Mental He vices Today a row

Experience iving care

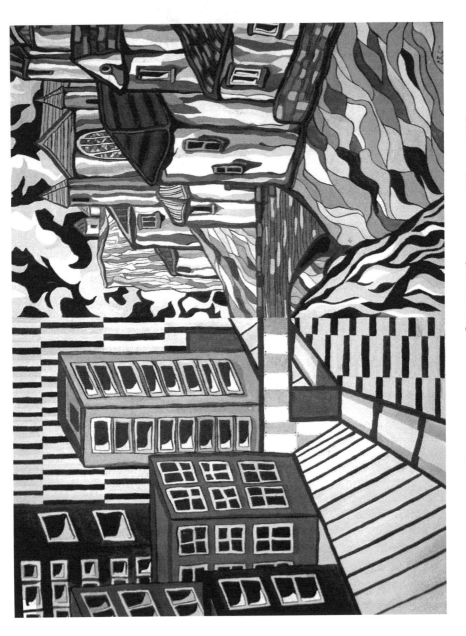

Steel & Stone by Rebecca Convery © 2007. Oil on canvas, 75cm × 100cm.

Mental Health Services Today and Tomorrow

PART 1

Experiences of providing and receiving care

Edited by

CHARLES KAYE

Mental Health Services Consultant

and

MICHAEL HOWLETT

Director, The Zito Trust

Radcliffe Publishing
Oxford • New York

Radcliffe Publishing Ltd
18 Marcham Road
Abingdon
Oxon OX14 1AA
United Kingdom

www.radcliffe-oxford.com
Electronic catalogue and worldwide online ordering facility.

British Library Cataloguing in Publication Data

A catalogue record for this book is available from the British Library.

ISBN-13: 978 184619 185 5

Typeset by Pindar New Zealand (Egan Reid), Auckland, New Zealand
Printed and bound by TJI Digital, Padstow, Cornwall, United Kingdom

Contents

Preface

The progenitor of this book was a survey we carried out into the status, including successes and failures, of England's mental health trusts. We describe the origins and outcomes of that survey in our Introduction. The questions posed by the survey – and the absence or incompleteness of answers on key topics – convinced us that a more extensive treatment was appropriate. But how should we go about that?

We wanted to look forward to trace and anticipate change in mental health services and to try to assess the impact both of developments in the field of care and treatment and of the implications of new organisational change. But we sought to achieve this not principally by our own knowledge and analysis, but by turning to those involved in services at all levels – to draw upon their experience to give a fuller picture of today and to help sketch in tomorrow. It was important to us to balance academic scrutiny with personal involvement, to reflect national trends and local endeavours.

Thus, for example, we deliberately juxtaposed a personal account of one man's journey through mental illness against the emergence of a new national initiative which will affect the whole country involving the treatment of hundreds of thousands of individuals at a cost of millions of pounds. It is our own view that to fail to value the reality and validity of personal experience when reviewing the pattern of care is the equivalent of building without foundations. The essential touchstone of successful care and treatment is the effect on individuals; too often, in our experience, the management of mental health services focuses on targets and totals and loses sight of its responsibility to users, carers and staff. A welter of slogans, strategies, brands and initiatives can fail to describe what happens to patients in the sub-standard psychiatric intensive care unit, to the individuals who fall between the compartmentalised services, and to the ill and inarticulate who can be shoehorned into predetermined patterns of services for the convenience of the system or the neatness of the organisation.

Consequently we have looked for detailed scrutiny – and one which reflected what users, practitioners and academics observed and experienced. Using the themes and topics identified by our survey, we commissioned chapters from a wide range of contributors asking them to describe the present and to anticipate and predict future changes, opportunities and threats. We chose contributors on the basis of their expertise and directed them towards key topics that we considered central to the future provision of care. We took pains to achieve the balance we have described. We also wanted to reach out beyond the island to take some soundings from mainland Europe. What is happening elsewhere? How might that affect our future here? Just as some contributors describe very personal experiences, so others explore a quite uncertain future, speculating and extrapolating.

From all our contributors we looked for a reasoned balance between success and problems, between observation and prophecy. We have avoided both the fatuously optimistic and the doomsayers. Above all, we invited them to 'write it as they see it'. We feel that the resulting collection of accounts gives a wide-ranging and valuable assessment of mental health services in England today.

We did, however, make a conscious editorial decision not to explore forensic mental health services in any depth (although we do refer in Part 2 to the funding of this part of the service). One of the seminal works in the field (*Forensic Psychiatry*, edited by Gunn and Taylor, first published in 1993) is being extensively revised and will be published in 2009.

Our goal in assembling and editing these contributions has been to depict realistically the current service, to outline sympathetically its features and flaws and to suggest where future emphasis needs to be placed, both locally and nationally, to make significant improvements and, above all, to make it more responsive to the needs of users and carers.

We have arranged the material in two parts. Part 1 focuses on experiences of receiving and offering care and on the realities of providing services at a practical and local level. It is an account of frontline life in today's mental health services. In Part 2, we take much more of a helicopter view, reviewing policy and practice from national and European perspectives. The two approaches are, of course, interdependent and interlinked and both should be explored.

Our own chapter in Part 2, 'Harnassing the flow', concentrates on what seem to us the most important messages that our survey highlights. Our contributors have identified a number of specific proposals that we consider would significantly improve the current service. One curious phenomenon that struck us in the task was that for all the national target-setting, organisational reshaping and the deluge of guidance, mental health services seem to lack personality; it is, in some contexts, closely defined but as a national player, curiously amorphous and passive. It would be encouraging to think that as Foundation Trust status becomes the norm, attention could be paid to the goal of creating an effective lobby representing all those personally involved in the service, a lobby that could help bring about change based on the evidence and experience of those directly involved.

Perhaps these books and their contributors might represent a significant step towards that destination.

Charles Kaye
Michael Howlett
April 2008

List of contributors

Lord Victor Adebowale joined Turning Point as Chief Executive in 2001. Turning Point is the UK's leading social care organisation working with people facing a range of complex needs including substance misuse, mental health problems and learning disabilities. Victor began his career in local authority estate management before joining the housing association movement. He worked with Patchwork Community and Ujima housing associations. He was Director of the Alcohol Recovery Project and Chief Executive of youth homelessness charity Centrepoint. In 2000, Victor was awarded the CBE for services to the New Deal, the unemployed and homeless young people, and in 2001 he was appointed a People's Peer.

John Adlam is Principal Adult Psychotherapist at Henderson Hospital Services and Group Psychotherapist at St George's Adult Eating Disorders Service, Springfield Hospital in London. He is an honorary lecturer in Forensic Psychotherapy at St George's University of London and also lectures for the postgraduate certificate programme in Working with People with Personality Disorder at the University of East London. John is a member of the Tavistock Society of Psychotherapists and Treasurer of the International Association for Forensic Psychotherapy.

Alastair Campbell was political editor of the *Daily Mirror* and Assistant Editor of *Today* before becoming spokesman and press secretary for Tony Blair in 1994. With Labour's election victory in 1997 he became the Prime Minister's Chief Press Secretary and Official Spokesman. In 2001, following Labour's second landslide election victory, he became Tony Blair's Director of Communications and Strategy. He resigned in 2003 and concentrates on lecturing, writing and raising funds for the Leukaemia Research Fund (www. lrf.org.uk). His book, *The Blair Years*, was published in 2007.

Neil Carr is Chief Executive of South Staffordshire NHS Foundation Trust, having spent nearly thirty years in the NHS. After training as a mental health nurse he held a number of executive posts in mental health and learning disability services. He has supported service user-led initiatives, better integration of primary and secondary care services and new ways of working. Neil is a strong advocate for improved educational provision for those delivering mental health services. In 2005 he was awarded an OBE for services to healthcare. He is a Fellow at Staffordshire University and is currently collaborating with South Carolina Medical School and the School of Health in Denver, Colorado.

Mason Fitzgerald is the Trust Board Secretary of the East London and the City Mental Health NHS Trust and a lead on the governance and membership aspects of the Trust's application for Foundation Trust status. He is a qualified barrister and solicitor and was formerly the Trust's Consumer Relations and Legal Affairs Manager.

Caroline Hawkings is Senior Policy Advisor for Mental Health at Turning Point. Dual diagnosis is an important area of work as a significant number of people using Turning Point's services have co-existing mental health and substance misuse needs. Turning Point is currently undertaking a national Dual Diagnosis Good Practice Project, resulting in a handbook for practitioners, due out in the summer of 2007. Caroline is also co-author of the *Dual Diagnosis Toolkit*, a practical guide for professionals produced in conjunction with Rethink in 2004.

Rory Hegarty joined the NHS with over ten years' experience working in the voluntary and public sectors. He brought with him experience of running national media campaigns on issues affecting carers, consumers and older people and has provided freelance media awareness support and training to a number of voluntary sector organisations. He is keen to see NHS Trusts develop closer links with service users, schools and the voluntary and private sectors as part of its drive to deliver public health messages and campaigns.

John Holt is an artist, lecturer, curator and cultural activist. He studied Fine Art at Leeds College of Art. A career followed teaching in schools, colleges and finally Leeds University where he was lecturer in Fine Art, Art History and

Cultural Studies. He headed the MA Fine Art course whilst at Bretton Hall. He was Fellow in Art and Design at Loughborough University for two years and has exhibited widely as an artist. His work at Rampton Hospital led to the setting-up of Artists in Mind (AIM) in 2002, an active organisation working in the fields of art and mental health.

Michael Howlett graduated in Law from Cambridge University and, after a period of teaching, joined the therapeutic staff at Peper Harow in Surrey, working with emotionally damaged adolescents and young offenders. He worked for the national High Security Psychiatric Service with Charles Kaye before becoming Director of The Zito Trust in 1994 which is now based in Hay-on-Wye. He has contributed a number of articles and book chapters on mental health and community care policy.

Francis Josephs joined the Highfield Family and Adolescent Unit at the Warneford Hospital in Oxford in 1990 after a career in teaching, having been Head of English and then Head of Sixth at a comprehensive school in Oxford. In 1996 he was appointed teacher in charge of the school in the Unit, and then took early retirement in 2003 but stayed on as a part-time teacher until 2005. A few months later Francis came out of retirement to take up a post with the nursing team as a part-time Care Assistant, a post he currently holds.

Charles Kaye graduated from Manchester University and trained in hospital management with the King's Fund in London. He held a variety of management posts in the NHS before being appointed in 1989 Chief Executive of the national High Security Psychiatric Service. Currently he is involved in social housing and in the provision of homes and employment for young people. He was awarded an OBE in 1996. He has edited and written books on the arts in healthcare, the management of high-security services, and on race and culture in secure psychiatric settings.

Tony Lingiah commenced his professional career as a general nurse and later graduated with both first and higher degrees in Education. He has been a lecturer in healthcare for 25 years and was latterly senior lecturer in forensic mental health for Broadmoor Hospital. He set up Abbeyfield Lodge in 2001 and was the Clinical Manager there for five years.

Jenny McAleese qualified as a chartered accountant after reading Modern Languages at Oxford. Whilst employed in the private sector she was seconded to the NHS and then spent two years as a health sector management consultant, specialising in the Private Finance Initiative. She joined The Retreat in 1996 as Finance Director, becoming Chief Executive a year later. A former trustee of the Diana, Princess of Wales Memorial Fund, she is a lay member of the Finance Committee of the University of York and trustee of a small mental health charity. She also serves as an Associate Hospital Manager for the local PCT.

Baroness Molly Meacher is Chair of the East London and the City Mental Health Trust and a crossbench member of the House of Lords. She has been the Chairman of the Security Industry Authority and Deputy Chairman of the Police Complaints Authority. In the 1990s Molly worked in Russia for four years, advising the Russian Government on the development of a system to handle unemployment. She is the author or editor of a number of books on the benefits system, mental health and the tax system. She was actively involved in the development of the Mental Health Act 1983 and spent five years as a Mental Health Act Commissioner.

Nuala O'Brien has worked in communications in the health service for more than 15 years; first in high-security mental health services, then in the acute sector, before joining West London Mental Health NHS Trust in 2005. In making the transition from forensic to acute mental health services, she recognised both a willingness and a need to involve service users and their carers in active and meaningful debate about issues which affect their lives. The launch of the national SHiFT campaign to challenge stigma in mental health provided a natural platform for the work Nuala and her team have focused on in their work.

Helen Pelendrides qualified in medicine at Guy's Hospital Medical School in 1984, and completed a further three-year period of specialist general practice training. She then worked as a GP principal in an affluent North London suburb for 14 years, in a large multi-site practice serving approximately 11 000 patients. For the last three years she has been working in a much smaller practice of around 3500 patients in a more deprived part of London. Helen has a training role with overseas graduate doctors and is also a director of a GP out-of-hours co-operative in North London.

Andrew Rogers studied Humanities at St Andrew's University in Scotland. He was first diagnosed with schizophrenia at the age of 21 in his third year at university. He subsequently taught English in China and worked in financial services in Saudi Arabia.

Christopher Scanlon is a Consultant Psychotherapist in the Department of Psychotherapy at St Thomas' Hospital, London. He is also a group analyst and an educational and organisational consultant. He is an honorary lecturer in Forensic Psychotherapy at St George's University, London, and visiting tutor at the Tavistock and Portman NHS Trust and is a member of the teaching faculty at the Institute of Group Analysis and the Turvey Institute for Group Psychotherapy. He is an associate member of An Organisation for Promoting Understanding of Society (OPUS) and a trustee of The Zito Trust. He was formerly Consultant Psychotherapist and Training and Consultation lead for Henderson Hospital Services in Surrey, and Course Director for the postgraduate certificate programme in Working with People with Personality Disorder the University of East London

Debbie Singh is an independent researcher, service evaluator and evidence analyst working with universities, charities, the NHS and local authorities services to improve health and social services. She is Chair of the NHS Centre for Reviews and Dissemination Expert Oncology Panel, Senior Associate at the University of Birmingham Health Services Management Centre, Evaluation Lead for the Surrey and Sussex Transforming Chronic Care Programme, Evaluator for the National Childbirth Trust, editor of various health journals, and service evaluator for numerous Primary Care Trusts and Strategic Health Authorities. Her main interests are in service development, improving access to services, and involving service users in design, implementation and evaluation.

Sharon Squires qualified as a registered mental nurse and has 31 years of accumulated experience of practice and management in different specialities, both locally and working at national level. She has enjoyed a variety of different positions and roles, including ward manager, team leader, practice development lead, change manager and Modern Matron where she currently works with older people. She has a keen focus on driving forward improvements in service provision and quality of care for all service users and staff.

Deborah Thompson completed her general nurse training in 1988 in Norfolk and her mental health training in 1991 in Lancashire. She moved to Nottinghamshire Healthcare in 1991 as a deputy ward manager. She has worked within the Older Persons directorate for the past 15 years and has recently been appointed the Modern Matron for Older Peoples Services for North Nottinghamshire.

Andrew Wetherell has worked in the mental health service user movement since 1994. His work has included developing self-help support initiatives and managing advocacy services. In 1997 he chaired the United Kingdom Advocacy Network and was a member of the Government's Independent Reference Group. He then became responsible for service user participation at Ashworth, Broadmoor and Rampton high-security hospitals. He has worked with the Hamlet Trust, developing service user initiatives in Central and Eastern Europe. He currently runs a mental health training and development consultancy with his wife, Roberta. Andrew is an associate trainer with The Sainsbury Centre for Mental Health.

Roberta Wetherell is a founder member and former national co-ordinator of the UK Advocacy Network, and founder chair of the European Network of Users and Ex-Users in Mental Health. She was a member of the NHS Executive's Mental Health Task Force User Group and has sat on committees advising the UK Government and the European Parliament. She has published work in advocacy, in training packs and for The Sainsbury Centre for Mental Health, where she is an associate trainer. Roberta is also a Mental Health Act Manager in one of the large London boroughs.

Acknowledgements

The editors would like to thank the following for their invaluable support at various stages in the preparation of the book: Hilary Burch, Ella Chidgey, Mary Crawford, Margaret Cudmore, Alan Franey, Brenda Goddard, Deborah Hart, Vivien Norris, Malcolm Rae, John Wilderspin and Deborah Williams. They would also like to thank Radcliffe Publishing for commissioning the book and Gillian Nineham and her colleagues for their editorial guidance and advice throughout.

Excerpt from 'Waking in the Blue' from *Collected Poems* by Robert Lowell, © 2003 by Harriet Lowell and Sheridan Lowell. Reprinted by permission of Farrar, Straus and Giroux, LLC.

Excerpt from 'The Second Coming' by WB Yeats. Reproduced with permission of AP Watt Ltd on behalf of Gráinne Yeats.

The editors would also like to thank the artists from Artists in Mind and Core Arts for contributing their work to the book. Both organisations exist to support and promote the artistic and creative abilities of people who experience severe and enduring mental health problems. For further information visit: www.artists-in-mind.org.uk and www.corearts.co.uk

to Hilary and Mary

I am: yet what I am none cares or knows,
My friends forsake me like a memory lost;
I am the self-consumer of my woes,
They rise and vanish in oblivious host,
Like shades in love and death's oblivion lost;
And yet I am, and live with shadows tost.

JOHN CLARE 1793–1864

(From 1837 until his death, Clare was a patient in asylums in Essex
and Northamptonshire.)

After a hearty New England breakfast,
I weigh two hundred pounds
this morning. Cock of the walk,
I strut in my turtle-necked French sailor's jersey
before the metal shaving mirrors,
and see the shaky future grow familiar
in the pinched, indigenous faces
of these thoroughbred mental cases,
twice my age and half my weight.
We are all old-timers,
each of us holds a locked razor.

ROBERT LOWELL 1917–77

(From 'Waking in the Blue', describing one of Lowell's stays at
McLean Hospital, Belmont, Massachusetts.)

Introduction

CHARLES KAYE and MICHAEL HOWLETT

AIMING FOR EQUALITY

One consistent reality throughout the history of the National Health Service (NHS) has been that mental illness and its treatment has come a poor second to those services devoted to treating acute (physical) conditions. The reasons for this are understandable: negatively, mental illness has been a disturbing shadow, threatening and apparently unpredictable; positively, the treatment, and perhaps care, of sick children, cancer, defective joints, etc., has an obvious urgency and appeal. This established, although not formally recognised preference, has been a leitmotiv in healthcare provision throughout our post-Bevan era. Attempts have been made to rectify this imbalance: the stand-alone psychiatric hospitals, with their own management committees, were in the 1970s integrated managerially – although not clinically – with local acute hospital services. Again more recently the deinstitutionalisation of psychiatric practice from the 1980s onwards – spurred equally by better medication and scandal – was a re-evaluation of priorities as well as a reconfiguration of care.

But as we entered the 21st century, with new definitions of the NHS involving commissioning, providers and contestability, it was clear that further change in the mental health service was in prospect.

Four key themes (there were others but these predominate) set the scene.
➤ A widespread conviction that while the refocusing from institutional care had largely succeeded as far as the dissolution of the large psychiatric hospitals was concerned, it had failed to provide an effective complementary network of community care. Evidence for this may have been mixed, ranging from vagrancy to violence, but the national

1

consensus was failure. As Frank Dobson, Secretary of State for Health, put it:[1]

> 'Care in the community has failed. Discharging people from institutions has brought benefit to some. But it has left many vulnerable patients to try to cope on their own. Others have been left to become a danger to themselves and a nuisance to others.'

➤ An intense national effort by the Department of Health (DH) to set national standards for healthcare and performance in virtually every dimension and direction – targets, modes of delivery, priorities, staffing. Above all, the NHS had to be *managed*: if the doctors, nurses and local managers could not deliver, then central government was prepared to tell them how to do it – and to critically monitor their progress.

➤ The preparation for the full implementation of the commercial culture within the NHS. The aim of this would be to abandon the 1940s monolithic paternalistic colossus, which seemed from the centre inefficient and ungovernable, and to create a market where providers competed for customer-patients under the watchful eye of the Whitehall umpire and paymaster. This movement has had various phases but has been a consistent drive within the actions and policies of both governing political parties over the past 20 years (although it has yet to find acceptance with the majority of NHS staff).

➤ The emerging awareness at a national and local level that the voice of the patient (more usually termed 'service user' in mental health) should have significance in the evolution and management of current and future services. Alongside this voice, there would also be choice – the reciprocal right of all customers.

Within those themes was blended a significant organisational change. Where for the past 25 to 30 years, mental health services had been deliberately brought within the 'acute' environment to end isolation and abolish the ghetto, now the way forward was to create specialist organisations which would focus on mental healthcare (and to a lesser extent on learning disability – a combination which echoed a long-standing confusion still not resolved). So the DH published its guidance for the new look in the NHS Plan of 2000 and a new national mental health service began, modestly, to emerge.

TAKING THE TEMPERATURE

Predictably this change, while it convulsed the world of mental health service workers, failed to attract significant national interest. As so often, mental health, and illness, was of little consequence unless it manifested itself in florid deviance and public horror. However, to those involved and keenly interested in mental healthcare, this set of changes – in national philosophy and local delivery – was both fascinating and crucial. Would it herald real change (as opposed to expensive re-labelling) and, if so, how would that change be demonstrated? Asking those questions, we decided in 2005 that it would be valuable to take soundings nationally to assess how the new specialist Mental Health Trusts were progressing and how they felt they were measuring up against the Government's targets and aspirations. To achieve this, we devised and despatched a questionnaire to all 84 Trusts that were then providing mental health services: that number included 14 Trusts who had formed a partnership with the relevant local authority for the joint provision of some services, and 18 Primary Care Trusts (PCTs) who continued to fulfil the dual roles of commissioner and provider, a gap-straddling posture that national policy will soon make impossible – despite any local resistance.

Our detailed findings and a full summary of the results are set out in the report *Today and Tomorrow*, published by The Zito Trust.[2] As outlined in our executive summary, the following key topics and concerns emerged – these arose from the Trusts' responses and reflect what a number of the providers were then experiencing. The overall picture we described thus:

> We have discovered wide variations in terms of size, demography, financial stability, management style and quality of service. Our report shows that while there are many examples of good practice, there remain a number of key concerns which raise fundamental questions as to whether mental health services in their current state can realistically commission and provide the level and quality of care set out in the Government's NHS Plan, National Service Framework for Mental Health and proposed new legislation. There are clear indications that the new configuration of mental health services is making only limited progress towards providing high-quality, user-centred services.

We identified seven key areas where Trusts were registering significant difficulties or slow progress.

➤ The annual cost of mental illness in England and Wales is estimated to be £77bn, more than the £60bn annual cost of crime. At a time of high funding levels generally, mental health services are not receiving an adequate or appropriate share of resources and their ability to develop is limited. They continue to lose out to acute hospitals. Many Trusts face budget deficits and are being forced to withdraw key services.

➤ Many Trusts face difficulties in recruiting and retaining good qualified staff. The vacancy rate for psychiatrists is 11%; for nurses it is 3%. Over 10 000 new staff are needed across the board. Mental health is not a popular field in which to work. Current services are under pressure and improvements to services are at risk.

➤ Considerable demands will be made on mental health services through the requirements of the Mental Health Act 2007. The requirement to develop new services and recruit appropriate staff cannot currently be met. One-third of Trusts have not yet fully implemented the Care Programme Approach introduced in 1991. Only 25% of Trusts have a full out-of-hours referral and support service. Bed occupancy rates are often in excess of 100%.

➤ Mental Health Trusts and PCTs are subject to an unreasonable and counter-productive regime of inspections by a large number of different bodies. One Trust quoted 96 different standards which have to be met. This continued emphasis on inspection and national target-setting absorbs scarce resources and significantly hampers Trusts as they try to develop their services.

➤ There is now an emerging second wave of reorganisation within and between Mental Health Trusts and PCTs. This includes applications for NHS Foundation Trust status. This second wave is of doubtful value and diverts attention and resources from key service objectives.

➤ There is evidence that some Primary Care Trusts do not demonstrate sufficient expertise or interest in expanding Mental Health Trusts and helping them to lift standards and expectations.

➤ Commendable efforts to involve users and carers are unfocused and unless they are properly directed will lead to misunderstanding and frustration.

Interestingly, a current ongoing survey[3] of Mental Health Trust chief executives again reflects many of the same concerns, particularly in the areas of Care Programme Approach (CPA) implementation, low confidence in commissioners and a preoccupation with reorganisation (Foundation Trust status).

Tempting as the Cassandra role was, we also willingly reported a great deal of success and enthusiasm across the country. We set out in the report the achievements that the Trusts themselves identified. They could be grouped in three principal areas.

➤ **Policy and process**
Trusts felt that they had established a vision of the future with clear priorities, that they were making good progress towards national targets and that they had agreed models for local services. Others had agreed a users' charter and adopted and launched diversity programmes.

➤ **Buildings and facilities**
Many Trusts featured this area of activity, identifying it as a speedy way in which to make improvements. Estate strategies had been developed, existing premises improved and new buildings commissioned – a number through Private Finance Initiative (PFI) deals. A number of Trusts described the closure of institutional-based facilities and the redistribution of resources for a new shape of service.

➤ **Improvements to infrastructure**
New management structures had been devised and implemented, financial balance achieved, staff morale improved and sickness absence reduced. A number of Trusts had integrated services with their social services counterpart. Some had improved their 'star' ratings.

These were examples: obviously not all Trusts claimed the same successes – and, of course, much was process-focused since most were new organisations establishing themselves.

PROBING MORE DEEPLY

The material we gathered, our own analysis and the comments our report attracted when published, indicated to us that a further examination of the contemporary mental health scene was required. Our 'snapshot' had given the new Trusts an opportunity to speak frankly, had ranged over the positives and negatives, the gains and the gaps. We were aware, however, that this was a developing picture; more features were becoming clearer and a one-off survey was not able to do full justice to a national pattern. Thus, as we describe, our books came into being.

REFERENCES

1 Department of Health. Press release 98/311. London: Department of Health; 1998.
2 Kaye C, Howlett M. *Today and Tomorrow: better services for mental health?* Hay-on-Wye: The Zito Trust; 2005.
3 Health Service Journal. Barometer. *HSJ.* 2007; **1 Mar:** 21.

CHAPTER 1

Honesty without discrimination

ALASTAIR CAMPBELL

The following is adapted from Alastair Campbell's speech to the 2006 Mental Health Media Awards, London. It is a frank discussion by a national figure of his own mental illness and the barrier it could have placed in the path of his career – were it not for an enlightened employer!

I have a fair bit of personal experience of mental illness and I have a fair bit of experience, too, of media misreporting creating fear, prejudice, bigotry and hatred.

You are not the first media awards event to invite me. But you are the first I have accepted. Most media awards are self-serving back-slapping sessions not worth leaving the sofa for.

But this is an awards ceremony that I think can make a difference. The Mental Health Media Awards, now in their 13th year, are successfully used to challenge – challenge stereotypes, challenge complacency, challenge the media to think beneath the easy-to-reach surface.

And for all I might rail at a lot of our media output much of the time, it doesn't actually make that much difference. If people really believed all the media pundits said about Tony Blair, he would never have survived as long as he has. I remember during the build-up to the Hutton inquiry, when we had a near permanent media camp on our doorstep, one of our neighbours said to me, 'You do realise if we believed what they were all saying, you would never walk out your front door?' And she was right.

People find their own perspective.

But I think mental health coverage is different. It is an area where the coverage itself, far from challenging a stigma, can help reinforce it, and in a way that has a direct impact upon the way people with mental health problems feel, are perceived, and the opportunities they are denied for fairness and equality, not least in the workplace but also as they go about their daily lives in their communities. Often met not with understanding but abuse and fear. Three times more likely to be harassed. Four out of 10 employers saying they would employ someone with a mental health history –that leaves six out of 10 who wouldn't.

I was incredibly lucky. I had a pretty spectacular nervous breakdown in 1986. I was lucky above all because I had a supportive partner, who had seen it all coming but was unable to make me see it, and who stuck with me when many others wouldn't. I had a small group of close friends, probably smaller after the breakdown than before, because something like that does tend to separate out the real friends from the drinking companions. I remember Alex Ferguson once giving me his definition of a friend – someone who walks through the door as others are preparing to put their coats on. Spot on. I had a brilliant GP and have always been lucky on the medical support front. Unlike many, I have also been lucky in the workplace. At the time I was on *Today*, but the then editor of my old paper, the *Mirror*, told me that he would take me back once I had found my feet again. That was an incredible act of support and friendship, all too often not found in worlds as competitive as the national media.

I was lucky, too, because although it was the worst time of my life, certainly the scariest, over time I turned it into one of the best, a life-changing event that made me stronger, fitter, more focused on the things that really mattered.

And I know without that strength I would not have been able to do the job I did from 1994 to 2003. When Tony Blair asked me to work for him, I said, 'You do know about my breakdown don't you? You do know I had a drink problem? You do know I still get depression from time to time?' He said, 'I'm not worried if you're not worried.' I said, 'What if I'm worried?' He said, 'I'm still not worried.' I think that is quite an important signal for us to take on board – that if the Prime Minister can take that attitude, so should other employers, too. Coincidentally the Government today launched a new programme to improve understanding of these issues among employers.

Part of this is still about basic attitudes. People who suffer from depression are still more likely to call in sick with fake flu than to admit the truth. I know people with schizophrenia who have held down jobs successfully but who are convinced they would never have got them if they had been open. Surely it is better for everyone if we can be honest without being discriminatory? Some people who suffer from schizophrenia will never hold down a job. But many can and could.

And though the media does now cover issues like depression and anxiety reasonably well, one area where I feel little progress is being made is in the constant linking of mental illness and violence. Most mentally ill people are not violent. Yet their issues tend to be in the media only when they are. One in eight of all stories about mental health has an angle related to violence. That is not representative. All the space devoted to virtually every aspect of our lives – people obsessed, it would seem, with their looks, their own physical well-being – conventional health covered extensively, but so little about this area which affects one in four directly, and that means all of us indirectly.

I recently opened an NHS [National Health Service] medium secure unit for severe psychiatric cases, a public–private partnership near Burnley. Amazing building. Great facilities. Fantastic caring and committed staff. Innovative therapies. Really humbling to look at some of the artwork of the patients, for example. But as I said at the opening, the only time the public will ever hear of the place is if one of the patients goes missing or if one of them attacks a member of staff really badly.

I think our mental health services, staff and patients alike, are a fantastic resource of powerful, uplifting emotional stories – the sort of thing I thought the media was meant to be about – but the general impression remains overwhelmingly negative.

And that has a real impact. That's why so many people will not tell even friends and family about their illness. They frequently report that the barriers they face because of diagnosis have a bigger impact on their lives than the symptoms.

Eighty per cent of journalists say they have personal knowledge – themselves or friends or family – of someone with a mental illness. Yet by a similar margin they admit the reality of mental illness is not reflected, that the picture is way too negative.

So tonight is about celebrating the good and hoping in so doing that we can raise awareness and so challenge the bad. Things do change for the better. 'Bonkers Bruno locked up.' Remember that one in the *Sun*? Of course you do. Changed to 'Sad Bruno in mental home' by the later editions because of the immediate furore. Signs of progress. But still day after day we can see the link between illness and violence, and in broadsheets, TV and radio as well as tabloids.

When dealing with stories about cancer, this is all presented sympathetically as a problem for the patients. Particularly if talking about young people. I know this, in the work I do as chairman of fundraising for Leukaemia Research. But when it comes to mental health, it is presented as a problem for society. It is all about risk to others, not help to the patient. It is the same approach taken, say, to asylum seekers, drug abusers, antisocial youths. Problem people, not people with problems. Yet there are three times as many people with serious mental health problems as there are people with cancer. Worth a thought.

Challenging stigma and changing attitudes takes time. But it happens. Black people still don't get into our mainstream media as much as they should. But it used to be they were hardly there at all, unless as heavyweight boxers, sprinters or convicted criminals. That has changed. Take gay issues. David Cameron standing up and saying he supported the civic partnership laws Labour had brought in. His audience may have looked like they had swallowed a lemon but they will get used to it. And so with issues of mental health coverage, we should pocket the progress but work for more: challenge the media to use sufferers as well as experts, let them know there are stories of hope and recovery as well as stories of violence and despair. And let sufferers know that, too. I know from my own experience how it helps to know there are other people out there who have been to the brink and come back. I benefited from that when I was ill. And I know from the letters I had when I did something for Mind a few years ago, that it is worth putting your head above the parapet on this.

Of course when you do, you will get the odd newspaper go to the usual rent-a-quote political pygmies to generate a fake storm. But that is the stuff that doesn't matter a damn. What matters is if you can help shape a change in attitudes.

I remember on the day I resigned from the Government and it was wall-to-wall on telly. I didn't see much of it but my sons were watching at home, and when Fiona and I got home, I asked who had been on. A mix of politicos and journos, but the one that clearly made an impression was Anne Widdecombe. She said I had been a terrible influence on politics – well she had to say that I guess and might even believe it – but what struck the boys most was her saying she admired me for the example I set in recovering from a breakdown and going on to do a job that would itself test most people to breaking point. I was quite proud of that. It is kind of what I feel and why, as I say, I look back on what I call my 'mad period' as both the worst and best experience of my life.

My main diatribe against the media is that we have more space than ever but, it seems to me, less ability to handle really complex subjects. The combination of intense competition, negativity, trivialisation, obsession with celebrity, an explosion in outlets, 24-hour news constantly on the lookout for the next whoosh, programmes now only interested in making a splash, rather than genuinely illuminating an issue; it all means there are few places where complexity is dealt with. And then there are the ghastly reality TV shows, modern-day freak shows where for titillation and ratings celebrities, so-called, are created and the nation can gorge on the psychodramas they play out. Not a happy scene generally, which is why it is so important to praise the exceptions as represented here.

Another point, as someone whose background was in newspapers. It is quite something that this is the first time the awards have felt able to make any award to the print media. I hope it helps encourage others to handle the subject more seriously, more sensitively, and with a deeper understanding of the issues.

Mental Health Media does a good job in trying to change attitudes. Its work will only be done, in truth, when there is no longer a need for it to exist. When these awards join the self-serving back-slapping category, we will know that the job is done, and MHM can then be wound up. Sadly, that day is some way off.

So let us honour the good and remember the bad.

CHAPTER 2

Community teams: outreach and intervention

NEIL CARR

The movement to a community-based service has been far from smooth – initial attempts are now seen as failures. This is a description of a 'new look' community service – responsive, flexible and measurable.

INTRODUCTION

Although the idea and, subsequently, the practice of community mental healthcare has been widely embraced in the United Kingdom since the 1960s, it is now becoming clear that, for it to be effective, much more is required than merely locating services randomly within communities. To deliver services effectively it is essential that those commissioning, providing and evaluating healthcare and health improvement recognise the social, economic and political environments in which they practise and the impact they have on the overall health and well-being of individuals and communities.[1] The driving forces behind the 'decarceration' of mental health patients still persist and have supported the psychotropic revolution, the patients' rights movement, the choice agenda and the closure of crumbling psychiatric hospitals. However, controversy is rife both within and beyond mental health services as to the success or otherwise of community care. Recently there have been calls from both the public and the professions to reinstate places of safety in which people with mental health problems can find refuge and be kept separate from society. While neither politicians, nor the public, nor service users, nor healthcare professionals would wish to see a return to the kind of mental healthcare that prevailed pre-1960, there is a general anxiety about the best way to proceed.

Mental health services have traditionally suffered from a sense of insecurity, more so than other branches of healthcare. This impacts on those who provide the services as well as those who receive them. Reviewing the situation of mental healthcare at the end of the 19th century, Porter[2] concluded that while medical science had made great advances, knowledge of mental health and of the brain remained weak. This sense of a gap in the professional knowledge base inspired an enthusiastic search for new treatments and interventions, many of which were adopted throughout the 20th century on very little evidence as to their safety or effectiveness. Examples include insulin therapy, psycho-surgery, electro-convulsive therapy, behaviour therapy, cognitive therapy, psycho-social therapies, psycho-pharmacological interventions. Some were found to be useful; others fell out of fashion as speedily as they had come into favour. Reflecting on the 20th century, Wells-Thorpe[3] concluded that it was possible that health professionals in all branches of medicine were still doing more harm than good. Concerns about mental health services persist. There are many who find services helpful,[4] but what they find helpful and how it is helpful remain unclear and require more research.[5]

Since 1997, Labour governments have made neighbourhood and community renewal a focus for their health modernisation agenda, based on the belief that 'healthy communities' are a prerequisite for a successful society.[6] More than 95% of people with mental health problems are now treated in community settings by primary care personnel. The reality for many mental health clients, however, is that the 'community' is represented by a single carer – in many instances, an unpaid female relative. Appropriate and effective care and treatment for individuals with mental health problem remains uncertain. However services evolve, they must present to every client the possibility of recovery and hope for the future, and move away from reducing distressed and confused people to passive dependency on drugs.[7] In this chapter, I explore some of the ideas being implemented by teams across the country in order to provide more responsive services and discuss practices that appear to be gaining the approval of service users and their carers. The nature of community, aspects of helping relationships, integrating services and choice and autonomy are key themes.

However, before examining examples of what seems to be good community practice, I wish to argue that a much better understanding of the nature and constitution of contemporary communities is required before we can understand how best to care for people with mental health problems within them.

THE VARIABLE CONCEPT OF COMMUNITY

Critics of community care find that it is based on a number of questionable assumptions, including its underpinning by an agreed set of principles and values, and the beliefs that communities are willing to accept those who are deemed to be different and that people with mental health problems are able to draw on the reservoirs of social capital that exist within communities. Simply establishing community services does not help service users if no account is taken of the culture and resources of communities.

Social theorists, policy-makers and service users may try to define and work with notions of society and community; however, all of them are 'prisoners of meaning' in that they are both participants in and producers of social reality.[8] What is that social reality, and how does it affect those who initiate and deliver community care? Anderson[9] starts from the somewhat unpalatable premise that, throughout history, groups of humans have been inclined to divide people into categories so that their own group comes out on top. This 'ghettoising tendency' affects individuals who are deemed to be different from those who hold the power in the community. Such individuals are devalued and discredited. An 'us and them' culture discourages interaction. Even pointing out that individuals are thus excluded further reinforces the differences between people; 'inclusion policies' may of themselves be devaluing. What services are called, who delivers them, where they are located and how they are funded may all be part of a stigmatising process. Referring to people as recipients of welfare, charity or short-term services further increases the stigmatisation. What service users want is not expensive; it is to be heard and valued, understood and respected and supported to attain their aims.

In the United Kingdom, where fear of mental illness is deeply ingrained, uncoordinated attempts to integrate people with mental health problems into communities can face immediate implicit and explicit rejection.[10] McCollum[11] argues that people must be fully incorporated into social networks before they can derive benefit from the social capital that exists in the community. 'The fly caught in the spider's web is included, but victimised.' Good community support is about meeting needs but primarily about enriching lives. It goes beyond the mere provision of therapy and advocacy, drawing on the countless community associations where those who were once labelled as being in receipt of treatment, counselling, advice and protection are incorporated into a network of relationships around work, recreation, friendship, support and citizenship. Professional power is problematical in the context of community-based services.[12] When professionals define the problem, treat it and evaluate the efficacy of the treatment, clients become passive recipients of care. Until people who are defined as having problems are allowed to redefine those problems in their own terms, community care is nonsensical.

Black[13] and Hines and DeYoung[14] highlight how Western thinking has always considered macro interventions recommended by the state to be superior to the various types of support available at the micro community level. This flawed assumption has eroded the social coherence that once characterised communities and eaten away at social capital. Now that we have reached the limits of institutional problem-solving, we must once again explore the possibilities of communities which include the exiled, the disaffected and the marginalised.[15]

> We all know that community must be the centre of our lives because it is only in community that we are citizens. It is only in community that we can find care. It is only in communities that we can hear people singing. And if you listen carefully, you can hear the words: 'I care for you, because you are mine, and I am yours.

Vanier[16] comes to similar conclusions. He claims that spending excessive time on service development is fruitless without first getting to know the structure and culture of communities and so gain an understanding of where to site services, who the providers should be and what other provisions are needed. Stainback and Stainback[17] contend that care in communities should mean that everyone has a part to play in both their own support and supporting others; helping others fosters self-esteem, mutual respect and a sense of accomplishment. Community cannot exist if certain people are always the receivers of support and never the givers.

Turner[18] argues that creating supportive communities is problematic in the light of the rise of human rights legislation, the erosion of national identity, the limitations of healthcare organisations and new definitions of care. Kurtz[19] discusses loneliness, especially in big cities. People with mental health problems have a debilitating sense of loss of companionship, resulting in loss of energy, ambition and a sense of relevance. Community care needs to embody and move forward a social agenda based on restoring and enhancing feelings of self-worth and self-esteem. While research has been able to identify obstacles and provide some solutions, there still exists a considerable distance between what is needed to support community care and what currently exists.

Commenting on the rise of community care, Prior[20] warned that while deinstitutionalisation had proved problematic, 'transinstitutionalisation' could prove even more so. He was referring to the way in which people were being moved between institutions and services – health services, social services, prisons and voluntary organisations. As more than 95% of mental

healthcare is provided in primary settings, Prior recommended that:
➤ better community-based services should be developed
➤ issues of risk and vulnerability in the community should be addressed
➤ a move should be made towards greater accountability in services
➤ primary care should play a greater role in mental healthcare provision
➤ user involvement and the inclusion agenda should be given a higher
  profile.

Rogers and Pilgrim[21] found that services were not being delivered to maximum
efficacy. Fifty-two per cent of general practitioners (GPs) did not provide sufficient information to service users about their conditions and treatments and
rarely suggested alternatives to medication; they allowed little time for mental
health clients. Nazareth *et al.*[22] identified a reluctance to collaborate between
mental health personnel from secondary and primary care sectors, and at the
turn of the millennium, Faulker[23] concluded that service users needed better
information about medication, longer consultation times and to be treated
with greater respect by their GPs.

Weiller *et al.*[24] noted a worldwide trend to identify and treat mental
health problems in primary care, but observed that that at least five European
countries were ill-equipped to accomplish this. Recognising the poverty of
the infrastructure to support the delivery of mental health services in primary
care, the *National Health Service (NHS) Plan*[25] set ambitious targets to be met
within a decade:
➤ 1000 new graduate mental health staff to be recruited into primary care
➤ an extra 500 community mental health team workers to be recruited
➤ 50 early intervention teams to be created to support young people with
  psychoses
➤ 335 crisis resolution teams to be created
➤ assertive outreach teams to be increased to 220
➤ women-only services to be established
➤ 700 extra staff to be recruited to work with carers
➤ better services for prisoners with mental illness to be set up
➤ a care plan and key worker to be in place for every person with a serious
  mental illness leaving prison.

The *NHS Plan* suggested that the services most likely to improve the mental
health of communities were crisis resolution, assertive outreach and early
intervention teams and primary care and mental health promotion.

HELPING RELATIONSHIPS

As has been repeatedly demonstrated, it is often the quality of the relationship that a person with mental health problems develops with the persons caring for him or her that determines the success of treatment.[26] It is not, however, yet clear what exactly it is that service users find most helpful in relating to providers. From the start of his career in psychotherapy, Carl Rogers sought to establish what it is that clients find helpful in a therapeutic relationship. He found that clients were generally less focused on the types of therapy they were receiving or the experience and qualifications of the therapist, but more interested in certain qualities of the person providing the service. These qualities were often to do with courtesy and respect, such as being on time for appointments, not missing appointments, remembering the name of clients and what had taken place at previous meetings, being non-judgemental and optimistic that recovery could take place. More recently, Roth and Fonagy[27] replicated some of Rogers' work and found that clients still highly valued personal qualities of caregivers such as warmth, empathy, sincerity and genuineness. They also appreciated 'skilful qualities' which included persuasiveness, the art of conversation – such as knowing when to interject – neutrality, and the ability to compromise.

Skills	Qualities
• Being able to demonstrate knowledge and experience	• Being warm and welcoming
• Being efficient and organised	• Being interested and reassuring
• Avoiding distractions and interruptions	• Being a good listener
• Being able to hold the attention of the client	• Being optimistic and hopeful
• Having good interpersonal skills	• Being able to conduct purposeful consultations
• Having good assessment skills	• Being honest and respectful
• Not rushing to conclusions	• Being able to negotiate outcomes
• Being aware of related services	• Being able to acknowledge progress
• Involving clients in their own care	• Being able to acknowledge their own limitations
	• Being able to cope with disappointment
	• Having a good sense of humour

A number of service users, including Harvey,[28] have commented on the need to understand what is happening in people's lives while they are in contact with mental health services and what is most important to them at the time. People may be in the process of losing their jobs, their homes, their families and their sense of who they are; hence a good carer must be able to preserve clients' sense of identity and self-esteem. They must be able to identify what has meaning and purpose for a particular individual, their interests, skills and ambitions, and focus on what people can achieve rather than starting with the 'problem'. Helping relationships are founded on certain qualities and skills in the caregiver.

INTEGRATED SERVICES

People with mental health problems may face more challenges in their day-to-day lives than any other group of people with disabilities. Not only may they be disadvantaged in terms of education, language, income, housing and nutrition, but many also suffer from isolation and financial insecurity.[29] People with severe and enduring mental health problems are four times more likely to have cardiovascular illness than the general population, five times more likely to be diabetic and eight times more likely to have HIV or AIDS. As a group, they have higher rates of smoking, obesity and alcohol consumption, which in turn predispose them to other forms of ill-health. Recent studies suggest that as many as 69% do not have an annual health check.[30]

Their experience of mental health services may be unsatisfactory. Approximately 30% of referrals from primary care to specialist mental health services are inappropriate.[31] Up to a third of all admissions to acute wards are unnecessary. And as many as 75% of people in high-security hospitals don't need to be there. Forty-five per cent of patients in one medium-secure unit have been deemed to be inappropriately placed.[32]

Unemployment rates are high among people with mental health problems, and admission to acute services makes it more difficult for them to retain or find employment. It is estimated that currently only 24% of adults with long-term mental health problems are in work, the lowest employment rate amongst any group of people with disabilities. Approximately 40% of those admitted into psychiatric wards do not return to their previous jobs. A study conducted in Bristol found that 80% of people who were in employment on admission to hospital were unemployed one year later,[33] and a further study found[34] that the workplace in most western countries is not conducive to good mental health. It has been concluded[35] that much more could be done to provide psycho-social support for vulnerable individuals in the workplace. There are over a million people currently on Incapacity Benefit as a result of being mentally ill, costing the country £750 per person per month – a considerable financial burden.[36]

Community mental health services need to be identifiable and discreet, but the real challenge is to dovetail closely with existing services in local communities. Much more needs to be known about how vulnerable people can be identified, how services are best provided for them and by whom. Mental health problems are experienced in many different ways and people in distress approach a variety of services. If help is to be provided appropriately and quickly, good relationships must exist between such agencies as Citizens Advice Bureaux, the Samaritans, Primary Care, Social Services and Human Resources Departments in the workplace. Activities that ensure collaboration and communication between services include:

➤ holding regular meetings to ensure familiarity with each other's services
➤ sharing knowledge and information about health-related issues
➤ devising assessment schedules and protocols
➤ arranging joint supervision sessions
➤ carrying out joint research projects and evaluations of services
➤ holding regular meetings with service users and carers
➤ establishing joint positions between services to foster good communication.

It is generally accepted that the quicker people's access to interventions, the better their chances of recovery or avoiding relapse. Health visitors, midwives, practice and community nurses, and GPs, should have a good grounding in recognising and responding to mental health problems. The potential of school nurses to impact on the early identification of need and appropriate intervention is a matter that has received little consideration to date.

Properly functioning integrated services are able to respond quickly and effectively to need. This means being able to undertake a comprehensive initial assessment that includes mental and physical health, social, family and work situations, what support the person has, what his or her priorities are in terms of getting better, what inner resources they have to draw upon, and their carers' priorities. The involvement of occupational therapists should be much more prominent at every stage of the client's journey than it has been to date. For such assessments to become embedded in practice, team-building has to be a top priority. Each team should comprise or have access to medical, psychological, nursing and social work personnel and be able to draw on other services such as pathology, X-ray and health education.

While the composition and functioning of community-based teams demonstrate considerable variation nationally, there is evidence as to what constitutes best practice in terms of maximising efficiency and effectiveness:

➤ service-users must be given choice at every stage; they should be involved in devising their care plans and contributing to their own care
➤ there should be a single access point to mental health services for people with mental health problems

➤ the time between onset of condition and provision of effective treatment must be kept to a minimum

➤ a comprehensive assessment and risk assessment should be undertaken

➤ a combination of biological and psycho-social interventions should be pursued

➤ treatment should be provided in the least restrictive setting and low dosage of medication should be preferred

➤ the person's social network and functioning should be maintained

➤ an appropriate key-worker should be selected to whom the client can easily relate

➤ a programme of engagement and psycho-education should be commenced

➤ a relapse prevention plan should be devised

➤ clients should participate fully in their own care and treatment.

COMMUNITY TEAMS

Crisis Resolution, Assertive Outreach and Early Intervention services that are well configured, comprise highly skilled personnel and offer an individualised approach to people and their carers not only provide choice to suit individuals' needs, but can reduce admissions to inpatient care, reduce the number of people admitted on sections, and engage with voluntary organisations and other community-based resources. Teams should be aware of the vulnerable people in their areas and those who are likely to require services in emergency situations. This is especially important for Crisis and Assertive Outreach teams who should aim not just to manage situations, but to manage the person in the situation and to understand why certain people do not wish to engage with services. Good services get to know vulnerable people when they are well and able to make decisions about their future. In this way, when people become unwell, providers know what they would want if they were able to make decisions. Well-designed community services can cut the number of admissions to acute care, reduce medication levels, limit referrals to other services and promote self-management.

Nationally there are many examples of services identifying local community resources and engaging them for the benefit of people with all types of health problems. In South Staffordshire NHS Foundation Trust, an Arts of Health initiative has invited local musicians, writers, artists and craftspeople to meet regularly and share their work with services users and staff. The aim of these meetings is to demonstrate the range of talents active in the community, the enthusiasm of creative people and the benefits they derive from their arts.

The visiting artists are unanimous in agreeing that they derive a great deal from their involvement with people with mental health problems and find it rewarding that their creativity and imagination can be restorative of other people's health. The centre in which these meetings are held is also the venue for meetings where ex-service users come to discuss their experiences of mental illness, how they coped, how they collaborated with their carers and what they have learned from the experience of illness. These are very popular with past and present service users. They provide an opportunity for people with a history of mental health problems to examine their life and practise the skills of reflection and critical thinking. Although these activities have not yet been formally evaluated, anecdotal evidence would suggest that service users appreciate learning more about their condition and what they can do to prevent relapse. Defining problems, asking questions, listening to responses, exploring solutions, increasing empathy and learning to value the notions of hope and recovery are skills that can be acquired during these meetings. Clients are learning to utilise people and resources that exist in the community in order to improve their understanding of themselves and their condition, and to improve the quality of their lives.

While there are pockets of excellent practice such as the illustrations given above in all parts of the country, the research to establish exactly what aspects of these activities are helpful to clients and how they could be developed remains to be done. It is uncertain whether the apparently good effects of community-based activities are short-lived or have a long-term impact in terms of improving the well-being of people with mental health problems and preventing relapse. Trusts continue to establish community-based mental health services and activities as directed by government policy while having a poor evidence base to direct their efforts. In-depth evaluative studies are urgently needed to ensure that resources of time, money and providers' enthusiasm are appropriately channelled to achieve maximum impact on the lives of people with mental health problems.

THE MAINTENANCE OF AUTONOMY, INDEPENDENCE AND ESTEEM

Good services acknowledge the important role that clients and carers play in the delivery of care and treatment. In the past, patients and service users were passive recipients of care, expected to agree to whatever was decided on their behalf. This approach eroded people's confidence and autonomy until they became unable to make even the smallest decision for themselves. Institutionalisation was a process of social suicide in which a person's dreams, beliefs, values and personalities were lost in a mélange of routine assessments and non-individualised care and treatments. Although it is now accepted that people should be consulted about what they want and should be involved in their own care, the *causes* of their mental health problems may be unaddressed. As a consequence, they may receive good care, but still not achieve complete recovery and full participation in society. Services need to focus on more than symptom reduction; they need to try to create the conditions in which mental health problems are reduced by assisting people with education, occupational functioning, finding adequate housing, dealing with the criminal justice system, and attaining an improved quality of life. Individuals receive poor care because of the separation that so often exists between acute, social and voluntary services. Issues around social inequalities and exclusion leading to or exacerbating mental ill-health need urgently to be addressed even though resources will never match demand, and mental health services may find themselves at the mercy of politics and policies. The World Health Organization[37] has stated that 'there is no health without mental health', and this is as true in the UK as anywhere else in the world.

Regardless of the particular kind of mental health problems people experience, services should ensure that people have as much information as they require and are assisted in making decisions that are in their own best interests. Health promotion needs to be emphasised much more with clients than it has been to date and mental health personnel should be collaborating with schools, colleges and universities. They should be educated to recognise the early onset of their condition and how to take immediate steps to minimise its severity. They should be enabled to make choices about their treatment and know the consequences of not adhering to their treatment regimens. Service users know the people who know about them and who can support them and they should therefore be helped to remain in contact with their social and family support systems. They are the experts about their own lives and problems.

The greatest respect that can be shown to service users is to assist them to take responsibility for their own lives and recovery. Knowing about one's medication and about how diet and exercise contribute to general health maintenance are important, as is the opportunity to have one's physical health checked regularly. Information about training schemes and support groups available within their own communities and how to access them is important, as is assisting people with parenting skills so that they can play a full part as members of their families. People should be encouraged to join in religious services and activities if they have a faith, and in social activities that promote their sense of social identity. Clients need to maintain their contact with work if at all possible and this may mean negotiating with employers and providing support in the workplace. Family members and carers have to be recognised as vital to the recovery process and they should be assisted to acquire skills that enable them to observe, assess and intervene when the occasion requires. They need to be included in all decision-making around individuals' treatment and care and their unique knowledge of the person must be valued and drawn upon by healthcare providers. They can both spot early signs of relapse and report on improvements in a loved one's condition.

Powerful community services ensure that individuals don't feel alone or ignored in their communities. All services should be 'hopeful', encouraging clients to believe that they will get better – even if this does not mean a full return to normality – and that they will be able to learn to live with their disabilities and build on and extend their own coping resources. Faster access to appropriate care would be enhanced if all primary care personnel could signpost clients to services within the NHS, to social services, voluntary services, local support groups and other complementary services. The essence of integrated services is that clients can be directed quickly and appropriately to what they need, rather than their struggling on their own to find help at times when their mental and physical functioning is compromised.[38]

REFERENCES

1 Gale E, Grove B. The social context for mental health. In: Bell A, Lindley P, editors. *Beyond the Water Towers.* London: The Sainsbury Centre; 2005.
2 Porter R. *Madness: a brief history.* Oxford: Oxford University Press; 2002.
3 Wells-Thorpe J. *Healing by Design: feeling better.* London: Royal College of Physicians; 2003.
4 Department of Health. *Treatment Choice in Psychological Therapies and Counselling: evidence-based clinical guidelines.* London: Department of Health; 2001.
5 Sharfstein S. Healing power of relationships. *Psychiat Interpers Biol Process.* 2005; **68** (3).
6 Means R, Richards S, Smith R. *Community Care, Policy and Practice.* London: Palgrave; 2003.
7 May R. *Mental Health: 'You could say I am a mad psychologist'.* Accessed at www.bradford.ac.uk/health/research/cccmh/files/MadPsychologist.doc
8 Giddens A. *The Third Way and Its Critics.* Cambridge: Polity Press; 1998.
9 Anderson A. Inclusion and interdependence: students with special needs. *J Educ Christ Belief.* 2006; **10**: 43–59.
10 West M, Poulton B. A failure of function: teamwork in primary health care. *J Interprof Care.* 1997; **11**: 86–94.
11 McCollum A. Tradition, folklore and disability. In: Eisland N, Saliers D, editors. *Human Disability and the Science of God in Assessing Religious Practice.* Nashville: Abingdon; 1998; 167–86.
12 McNight J. *The Careless Society.* New York: Basic Books; 1995.
13 Black K. *A Healing Homiletic: preaching and disability.* Nashville: Abingdon; 1996.

14 Hines S, DeYoung C. *Beyond Rhetoric: reconcilation was a way of life*. Valley Forge, PA: Judson Press; 2000.

15 Putnam R. *Bowling Alone*. New York and London: Simon & Schuster; 2001.

16 Vanier J. *Becoming Human*. Mahwah, New Jersey: Pauline Press; 1998.

17 Stainback S, Stainback W, editors. *Inclusion: a guide for education*. Baltimore: Paul H Brookes; 2002.

18 Turner BS. The erosion of citizenship. *Br J Sociol*. 2001; **52**: 189–209.

19 Kurtz I. *Loneliness*. London: Penguin Press; 1983.

20 Prior L. *The Social Organisation of Mental Illness*. London: Sage; 1993.

21 Rogers A, Pilgrim D. *Experiencing Psychiatry: user's views of services*. Basingstoke: Macmillan; 1993.

22 Nazareth I, King M, Davies S. Care of schizophrenia in general practice: the general practitioner and the patient. *Br J Gen Pract*. 1995; **45**: 343–7.

23 Faulkner A, Payzell S. *Strategies for Living: a report of user-led research into people's strategies for living with mental distress*. London: Mental Health Foundation; 2000.

24 Weiller E, Bisserbe C, Maier W *et al*. Prevalence and recognition of anxiety syndromes in five European primary care settings. *Br J Psychiatry*. 1998; **173**: 18–23.

25 Department of Health. *The NHS Plan: a plan for investment, a plan for reform*. London: Department of Health; 2000.

26 Peveler R, George C, Kinmonth A *et al*. Effect of antidepressant drug counselling and information leaflets on adherence to drug treatment in primary care: randomised controlled trial. *BMJ*. 1999; **319**: 612–15.

27 Roth A, Fonagy P. *What Works for Whom? a critical review of the literature*. Guildford: The Guildford Press; 1999.

28 Harvey Z. Effective collaboration with users. In: Nolan P, Badger F, editors. *Promoting Collaboration in Primary Mental Care*. Cheltenham: Nelson Thornes; 2002.

29 Meltzer H. Further analysis of the psychiatric morbidity survey 2000. London: Social Exclusion Unit; 2003 (unpublished).

30 Laugharne R. Psychiatry in the future. The next 15 years: post-modern challenges and opportunities for psychiatry. *Psychiatr Bull*. 2004; **28**: 317–18.

31 Social Exclusion Unit. *Mental Health and Social Exclusion*. London: ODPM; 2004.

32 Glasby J, Lester H. *An Overview of the Evidence which is Driving the Agenda for Change*. Hospital Services, booklet 5 of Cases for Change: National Institute for Mental Health in England; 2003.

33 Fenwick P. A pathway to employment. *A Life in the Day*. 2003; **7**(1): 4–5.

34 D'Souza R, Strazdins L, Broom D *et al*. Work demands, job insecurity and sickness and absence from work. How productive is the new, flexible labour force? *Aust NZ J Public Health*. 2006; **30**: 205–14.

35 Niedhammer I, Chastrang J, David S *et al*. Psychosocial work environment and mental health. *Int J Occup Environ Health*. 2006; **12**: 112–19.

36 London School of Economics. *The Depression Report*. London: The Centre for Economic Performance's Mental Health Policy Group; 2006.

37 World Health Organization. *Mental Health Declaration for Europe*. Geneva: WHO; 2005. Available at: www.euro.who.int/document/mnh/edoco6.pdf.

38 McGorry P. Evidence based reform of mental health care. *BMJ*. 2005; **331**: 586–7.

CHAPTER 3

Homelessness and disorder: the challenge of the antisocial and the societal response

CHRISTOPHER SCANLON and JOHN ADLAM

We begin with a discussion of the psychosocial concepts of 'homelessness', 'dangerousness' and 'disorder' and then seek to redefine and relocate both from the internal world of the individual sufferer to the psycho-social 'dis-memberment' associated with what we have called the 'unhoused mind'. We then explore the complex reciprocal relationship between the 'ordered' and the 'dis-ordered', the social and the anti-social, and consider some possible implications for individual workers, staff teams and organisations who are tasked with attempting to house or otherwise to accommodate such people. We conclude with a challenge for policy-makers to reframe the philosophical basis of their approach to the societal duty of care.

INTRODUCTION

The premise of this chapter is that despite considerable attention over recent years being addressed to the problems of anti-social people, much of it reviewed in this volume, there remains a group of people who steadfastly refuse to be included. Further, it is our contention that even if the best efforts of our most experienced workers were channelled to address these problems, which is rarely actually the case, there would always remain a group of people who would refuse to play the game and would resist all efforts to bring them 'in from the cold'. Whether they be dangerous people who present a risk to others, homeless people with complex needs who refuse to be settled, people with severe eating disorders who refuse to eat (or stop eating), people with drug and alcohol problems who refuse to stop damaging themselves through dangerous addictions, recidivist offenders who refuse to be corrected, or disaffected young people who refuse to be educated, there will always be people who will continue to refuse.

We further contend that all zero tolerance mental health and social policy directives that optimistically, or cynically, envisage a future when all such people will be 'socially included', essentially involve a dangerous and stubborn refusal to face up to the reality of these problems: a denial of their essential complexity and chronicity. It is dangerous because, no matter how 'politically correct' the policy, or how sophisticated the needs assessment tools, such belief systems are setting up to fail not only socially excluded people but also those workers charged with trying to reach out to them, and in their failing exacerbate the sense of exclusion and disaffection. The ubiquitous problem is how to relate to the refusal that is at the heart of these difficulties and it constitutes one of the major challenges facing all mental health, social care and criminal justice agencies.

THE DIOGENES PARADIGM?

In an earlier published article we explored links between homelessness and dangerousness, considered as states of mind as well as of body, and complex and severe personality disorders.[1] We offered, as a paradigm for the societal as well as clinical difficulties inherent in reaching out to the difficult-to-reach individual, the story of Diogenes of Sinope, the Cynic, who 'holed himself up' in a barrel in the main square in ancient Athens, and of his encounter with Alexander the Great, the most powerful man in the world. Asked by Alexander if there was anything he could do for Diogenes, the latter replied from his barrel, in terms familiar to any outreach worker who has knelt down alongside a homeless person's 'bash': 'Yes there is – you can step aside because you are blocking my light.' Diogenes' Cynicism was to refuse accommodation from societal systems that he regarded as fundamentally untruthful. For example, when seen carrying around a torch in broad daylight, he explained he was in search of 'one honest man'. He was known as 'Diogenes the Dog', which animal was strongly associated with shame in ancient Greek culture; and he would also express something of the shamefulness of his unhoused state by masturbating in his barrel. When challenged, he is supposed to have said that 'he wished it were as easy to relieve hunger by rubbing an empty stomach'.

Our observation has been that teams working with the modern-day Diogenes – with the homeless, the dangerous or the disordered – find themselves torn between one impulse to coerce them out of their places of refuge and into a proper accommodation and an opposite impulse to wash their hands of them and leave them out in the cold. The former case is often associated with an over-use of statutory powers, such as mental health legislation – whilst the latter case is often associated with an under-use of such powers. Our hypothesis is that organisations often struggle to understand the needs presented to them because concepts like 'successful resettlement', 'safe and secure disposal', 'proper accommodation' and other ideas about what constitutes a positive outcome are predicated upon the *workers'* experiences of having 'housed' and 'secure' states of mind, rather than upon any particularly methodical inquiry into what the *client* might actually understand by feeling safe.

Our hypothesis is that homelessness, dangerousness and disorder, when viewed from this perspective, could be seen as both symptom and communication of unhoused and dis-membered states of mind. For example, many in these overlapping categories of outsiders – labelled 'untreatable', 'unreachable' or 'unteachable' by mental healthcare, social care, criminal justice and education services – would also regard themselves as such, and so hold themselves outside the boundary of any organisation which tries to help them. They would not readily see themselves as 'clients' or 'service users', still less 'patients'. They then refuse to comply with related expectations about how they should present, and in so doing challenge and thwart our best efforts to assume the role of carer.[2,3] In a profound sense such people are both psychologically 'unhoused' and psycho-socially 'dis-membered' and further, like Groucho Marx, would not be a member of any club that would offer them membership.

Thus although the refusal of the unhoused to be accommodated may be regarded as cynical, our view is that many of the initiatives to get them back into 'productive citizenship' are, taken collectively (and we cast no aspersions on individual practitioners, clinicians or policy-makers), also deeply cynical – albeit at a more subtle but often no less ruthless or (structurally) violent level.[4]

INTENTIONALITY AND TREATABILITY

At the centre of this difficult relationship between the chronically unhoused, the dangerous and disordered, and so-called normative society, is the issue of *intentionality*. A powerful voice within the wider social system complains that some of these anti-social individuals who refuse to be included, and so hold themselves outside of normal societal rules, are doing so intentionally.

They are choosing to be outside and therefore we need not think about their needs. Rather than being seen as traumatised through experiences of poverty, deprivation, neglect and abuse, their anti-social stance is construed to be delinquent, deviant or offensive.[5] The impulsive societal response to this is then to 'lock 'em in', 'lock 'em out', 'throw 'em out' or 'lock 'em up'.

For example, under successive Housing Acts and court rulings, persons found to have made themselves 'intentionally homeless' are denied housing. Or a troubled and troublesome tenant in a supported housing project is deemed to have 'deliberately' broken the rules and so is 'asked to leave'. This dynamic is also played out in the education system in relation to how to deliver normative education to those who, for complex socio-economic reasons, stand outside such norms and maintain there is nothing of value to be learned.[6] It is also powerfully present in the way in which anti-social behaviour orders (ASBOs) are increasingly being used to criminalise those individuals and families in our society whose vulnerability and sense of social exclusion results in their feeling that they have nothing to gain by 'joining in'. At a more macro-political level the same dynamic is currently being played out with asylum seekers and economic migrants who face ever more complex and arduous scrutiny about whether or not, for whatever reasons, they are held to have rendered themselves stateless. In the politics of the body this dynamic is also played out in the response of parts of a healthcare system which seeks to deny healthcare to the obese, or to smokers, whose illnesses are seen as resulting from a lack of willpower, greed or laziness, rather than unhappiness, social exclusion or psychological dependency.

In the world of the personality disordered, people are often denied services because the self-harm, and/or violence, and/or self-neglect with which they present is held to be intentional.[7] The consequence for some people is that, out of a sense of violent desperation, they then go on to offend, or to harm themselves. Worse still, there is ample evidence that when 'healthcare' interventions are necessary they can often be more like 'revenge' or 'retaliation' or, at the very least, prejudice and discrimination.[8,9,10] Indeed, nearly 50 years ago Tom Main cautioned us all about such tendencies by stating:

> . . . the sufferer who frustrates a keen therapist [sic] by failing to improve is *always* [our italics] in danger of meeting primitive human behaviour disguised as treatment.[11]

DISTURBANCES OF 'GROUPISHNESS'

Viewed from this perspective, societal responsibility for these conditions can be seen as being bound up in a very complex interplay of reciprocal roles. As described above, one response is to seek to exclude the offending persons from society and put them behind walls or bars as if out-of-sight and out-of-mind. Alternatively, those with homes build ever longer and more heavily guarded perimeter walls to keep out and exclude the disordered, the disorderly and the dispossessed. Systems of care create ever more elaborate ways of excluding such people from our services and from our minds. The unhoused and the dis-membered are feared and pushed away because they threaten our idea of what it is to feel that we are in a secure and housed state of mind and members of so-called normal social groupings. However, such unhousedness and insecurity cannot be entirely split off and got rid of, precisely because there are parts of *all* our minds that remain insecure and unhoused.[12]

The *Diagnostic and Statistical Manual of Mental Disorders*[13] defines personality disorder as 'an enduring pattern of inner experience and behaviour *that deviates markedly from the expectations of the individual's culture*' (our italics), thus making clear that such disorders cannot be understood except in relation to the group at the edge of which the individual finds himself or herself. As such, we suggest that the psycho-social difficulty presented by this client group probably says as much about our anxiety as about theirs. Indeed operationally, if not diagnostically, we may well need to think about the problem as being that of an interpersonal disorder or at least what Bion[14] might have called a disturbance of 'groupishness', in which clients feel incompletely housed within, and dis-membered from, the structures and culture of their received familial, group and ethnic background.

Thus, the homeless, the dangerous and the disordered suffer from severe disturbances of groupishness, or dis-membership, and as we discussed in our previous work,[15] this experience is also accompanied by a profound sense of not being 'at home' in their body and in their mind. It is not surprising, then, that they so often present as being both literally and metaphorically 'scared out of their skins', 'at their wits' end', 'out of their minds' and 'beside themselves' with the painfulness of unbearable feelings. The question posed by the encounter with this state of unhousedness is how one might come to feel secure in the external social world when one's internal home/space is experienced as being chronically empty.

Bateman and Fonagy[16] show how this chronic emptiness links to the developmental failure to achieve a secure attachment and how traumatising processes can inhibit the development of mentalising capacity and reflective functioning, without which the emergent adult will remain in the sort of unhoused, dis-membered state of mind that we describe above. In terms of attachment theory, 'the secure base' is another way of saying that in ordinary development the experience of 'feeling at home' is linked to the experience of one's self as being housed in others' – usually parents' or the wider community's – minds. The likely outcome of secure attachment during childhood is a mind with a 'lived-in' feel, which can be valued and looked after. The homeless, the dangerous and the disordered, often traumatised by experiences of intrusion or abandonment in which the attachment figures were themselves the source of the danger, have been unable to develop the capacity to understand and process their own distress. In such cases, affectional and affiliative bonds have been snapped like so many nerve ends, never to recover the original contact points.

In this state of mind, such people seek to avoid 'being inside' anything, while all the time being held in the grip of a contradictory and equally strong wish to be known and inside the minds of others. Caught between these two poles of longing and fear, their life becomes an endless and painful oscillation between the intimacies and fear of the inside (claustrophobic anxiety) and the distances and sense of rejection and abandonment when on the outside (agoraphobic anxiety).[17] Such individuals live liminal lives: the doorstep, threshold, borderline and twilight become, in a sense, their only true homes, the only proper places where they can stand; 'unhousedness' has become their state of mind and 'dis-memberment' from the social body their way of life.

ON RE-MEMBERING . . .?

> The best lack all conviction, while the worst
> Are full of passionate intensity
>
> *WB Yeats, 'The Second Coming'*

Individual workers, teams and organisations working with these interpersonal dynamics inevitably find themselves caught up in related states of unhousedness or incohesion.[18,19] Some staff come to experience themselves as atomised and monadic, increasingly distanced and alienated both within themselves and from their colleagues; whilst others experience themselves as being in a gang-like state of mind.[20] The more these 'difficult people' resist and refuse attempts to put them 'inside' (which, of course is also a euphemism for being in prison), the greater the pressure on the worker. Thus a sort of dance is set up, in which the lead is constantly moving back and forth across a boundary characterised by the oscillating 'desire' of the worker and client respectively.

The possibility of a more empathic understanding is very easily replaced by workers' constant unconscious attempts to defend themselves and/or each other against the anxiety that emerges in the face of this refusal and rejection. Professional 'goods and services' are apparently exchanged but the net result is a zero sum game in which there is no movement and no growth. The irresistible force meets the immovable object and the organisation that was established to house traumatised and dis-membered people with unhoused minds becomes itself a traumatised organisation employing the services of dis-membered staff with increasingly unhoused minds.[21,22]

In this fragmented state, the kinds of group activities, staff meetings, supervision and training that would usually provide staff members with a sense of cohesion and personal identity become a source of tension and are avoided. In this state, any sharing of workers' experiential understanding of the pain of 'the would-be client', instead of being remembered, reflected upon and worked through within the group, is denied – as both clients and staff teams adopt an unconscious but secretly shared task that could be defined as the pursuit of a state in which all knowledge of all distress is to be forgotten and dis-membered from the body of experience.

In our experience, instead of remembering the pain of the homeless, the dangerous and the disordered and their own disturbed relationship to it, and often as a reaction to the real and apparent lack of conviction of the wider system of care, organisations in this state of mind can often find themselves taking up a rather macho positioning in a problematic identification with the socially excluded. The agency begins to see itself as 'lean and mean' and the staff become cast in the role of the hero, doing a dirty job under difficult circumstances in order to clean up somebody else's mess. They frequently see themselves as the people who like to say 'yes' when 'the system' has said 'no'. Often the dress and demeanour of staff is suggestive of the alienated outsider, and communicates a confusion of vulnerability and aggression which mimics rather than reflects the world of the clients. The communication is rooted in a wish to work what is for the most part a macho deception, based on identification, that 'I know what it is like to be you.'

In our experience, there is a concentration of such staff within some specialist teams, where widespread hostility towards mainstream statutory services, coupled with a problematic identification with the (oppressed) client group, often involves a flight into a spuriously gratifying war on authority as a reaction against those other agencies that are perceived as having been oppressive and excluding. A resultant 'none shall be turned away' attitude can then give rise to a highly politicised 'rights' culture, with a correspondingly diminished sense of professional role and responsibility in which the mantra becomes that clients must be given everything they demand – even as they violate the rights of others.

This tendency is, however, always oscillating with an alternative, equally dogmatic and authoritarian attitude, from other staff and/or other agencies who simply want to evict, expel or exclude troublesome individuals who challenge their ever more tentative grip on their personal and professional authority. The resultant divisions and splits within staff teams and between agencies then become sources of real conflict and disagreement that often become very difficult to 'manage'.[23,24] A typical reaction is that staff move quickly to complaining to or about 'the management' and 'the authorities', without seeing the extent to which their complaint is rooted in a problematic unconscious identification with the client, and that in so doing they may also be relinquishing their own self-management.

The actual managers and real authorities then find themselves confronted with parallel dilemmas. Either they identify with their workers' identification with the clients and agree that the enemy is without, or they accept the blame and recriminations and so have to 'field' the hatred and anger that comes with that position. In the absence of meaningful team cohesion, and in order to survive the workers' onslaught, the former course is often chosen, and the 'complaint' is then passed through the organisation without being digested and is shovelled onwards and upwards into 'the system'. This in return evokes the familiar 'lock 'em out' response from the wider system of care, and as a result the agency itself is experienced, in the parallel process, as being as troublesome as its patients; it is damned by association and the agency, like its clients, becomes un-housed and dis-membered from the wider system of care. At this point, of course, all have finally achieved the unconscious objective of forgetting what they are there to do. The primary task of remembering the grief associated with the clients' original traumas is replaced with an expression of a grievance. Sometimes the grievance is expressed as if on behalf of the clients, while at other times they are complaints about the clients expressed on their own behalf, but in both cases the original problem has been replaced by what Main[25] described as 'the ailment'. It is often at this point that serious and untoward incidents occur.

In outlining the above, however, we are *not* suggesting that individual staff members, or agencies, who get caught up in these dynamics are necessarily any more pathological than any other. We would no more ascribe intentionality to those caught up in these dynamics than we would to the clients, nor would we wish our hypotheses to be used in either direction as a basis for blame or recrimination. Rather, we are suggesting that the study of these dynamics, as part of an ongoing psycho-social 'culture of inquiry', could, with skilled facilitation, provide valuable information about the lived experience of the client group, their traumas and the societal roots of these traumatising processes.[26] Also, in common with Hopper,[27] we are suggesting that the processes that we have described are discernible in all organisations that work with very traumatised and difficult people, in difficult places, and that directors, managers and supervisors in such projects underestimate the power and ubiquity of these processes at their peril.

SOME CONCLUDING REMARKS

'For the poor always ye have with you . . .'

John 12:8

In this chapter we have outlined some of the dynamic processes emerging from working with difficult clients in difficult circumstances. We have suggested that it is very often the case that those people who do refuse to be included are also those who present the greatest danger – usually to themselves, but also to others. Yet our observations have been that such people also have very low social worth with a corresponding relative lack of investment, both in socio-economic and emotional terms, the result of which is that they are driven further to the edge. We would further observe that this tendency reflects the normative values of a world in which it is acceptable for the rich to get richer whilst the poor get poorer.[28]

We have suggested that ideas of psychic 'unhousedness' and psycho-social 'dis-memberment' might be useful ways of conceptualising the presenting difficulties of these clients as well as the complementary experiences of staff who find themselves working in these very difficult settings. We also have suggested the capacity of any organisation to offer a cohesive approach to care under such pressure is consequent upon the capacity of individual workers to become members of the teams within which they can feel housed, or think about the ways in which they remain unhoused, and within which they can establish formal ways of metabolising their experience of being exposed to the types of human misery that we are calling psychological unhousedness and psycho-social dis-memberment. Only then can they really begin the task of re-membering the traumatisation of the clients and so think clearly about the proper accommodation of their problems rather than submitting to the emotional and social desire to 'lock 'em in', 'lock 'em out', 'throw 'em out' or 'lock 'em up'. Our plea is for greater tolerance, understanding and interest in the lives of the homeless, the dangerous and the disordered who have found themselves on the borderlines of our deeply troubled society, and for a better informed debate between adult mental health, children's services, and the criminal justice systems about how to introduce the structural and cultural changes that will be necessary to support organisations and their staff to relate meaningfully to some of the most vulnerable members of our community in concerned and humane ways – whether they, or we, like it or not.

We would like to explore the possibilities of reclaiming from Diogenes his Cynicism with a capital 'C'. If it must be that 'the excluded always we have with us', then it would be cynical indeed to take this as a basis for indifference and inaction. But it might be Cynical in a healthier sense for us to question repeated, possibly manic attempts to wish away the complexity and chronicity of the problem by insisting on their inclusion, and instead to explore different ways of understanding both our difference and our kinship. To return to our paradigmatic tale, Alexander is reputed to have been so moved by his encounter with Diogenes as to have remarked: 'If I were not Alexander, I would be Diogenes'. Let us not suppose either protagonist to have been a happy man.

Acknowledgements: We would like to acknowledge the contribution of those who took part in the Governing Minds Conference in Oxford, March 2006, and the Tavistock and Portman NHS Trust's Social Policy seminar in October 2006, especially Jessica Evans from the Open University, Andrew Cooper from the Tavistock and Portman NHS Trust, Mike Rustin from the University of East London and Vickie Cooper from Sheffield Hallam University.

REFERENCES

1 Adlam J, Scanlon C. Personality disorder and homelessness: membership and 'unhoused minds' in forensic settings. *Group Analysis. Special Issue: Group Analysis in Forensic Settings.* 2005; **38**(3): 452–66.

2 Adshead G. Murmurs of discontent: treatment and treatability of personality disorder. *Advances in Psychiatric Treatment.* 2001; **7**(6): 407–14.

3 Norton K. Management of difficult personality disorder patients. *Adv Psychiatr Treat.* 1996; **2**: 202–10.

4 Gilligan J. *Violence: reflections on our deadliest epidemic.* London: Jessica Kingsley; 1996.

5 Ibid.

6 Maher M. Therapeutic child care and the local authority. In: Ward A, Kasinski J, Pooley J *et al.*, editors. *Therapeutic Communities for Children and Young People.* London: Jessica Kingsley; 2003.

7 National Institute for Mental Health in England. *Personality Disorder: no longer a diagnosis of exclusion.* Policy implemetation guidance for the development of services for people with personality disorder. London: NIMHE; 2003. Available at: www. nimhe.org.uk

8 Blom-Cooper L. *Report of the Committee of Inquiry into Complaints about Ashworth Hospital: volumes I and II*. London: HMSO; 1992. Available at: www.bopcris.ac.uk/bopall/ref23676.html

9 Kelly MP, May D. Good and bad patients: a review of the literature and a theoretical critique. *J Adv Nurs*. 1982; **7**: 147–56.

10 Lewis G, Appleby L. Personality disorder: the patients psychiatrists dislike. *Br J Psychiatry*. 1988; **143**: 44–9.

11 Main TF. The ailment. *J Med Psychol*. 1957; **30**: 129–45.

12 Foster A, Roberts VZ. *Managing Mental Health in the Community: chaos and containment*. London: Routledge; 1998.

13 American Psychiatric Association. *Diagnostic and Statistical Manual of Mental Disorders*. 4th ed. Washington, DC: American Psychiatric Association; 1994.

14 Bion WR. *Experiences in Groups*. London: Routledge; 1961.

15 Adlam J, Scanlon C. Op. cit.

16 Bateman A, Fonagy P. *Psychotherapy for Borderline Personality Disorder: mentalization based treatment*. Oxford: Oxford University Press; 2004.

17 Glasser M. Aggression and violence in the perversions. In: Rosen I, editor. *Sexual Deviation*. Oxford: Oxford University Press; 1996.

18 Adlam J, Scanlon C. Op. cit.

19 Hopper E. *Traumatic Experience in the Unconscious Life of Groups: the fourth basic assumption*. London: Jessica Kingsley; 2003.

20 Rosenfeld HA. A clinical approach to the psychoanalytic theory of the life and death instincts: an investigation into the aggressive aspects of narcissism. *Int J Psychoanal*. 1971; **52**: 169–78.

21 Adlam J, Scanlon C. Op. cit.

22 Hopper E. Op. cit.

23 Ibid.

24 Gabbard GO, Wilkinson SM. *Management of Counter-transference with Borderline Patients*. Washington, DC: American Psychiatric Press; 1994.

25 Main T. Op. cit.

26 Gilligan J. Op. cit.

27 Hopper E. Op. cit.

28 Gilligan J. Op. cit.

CHAPTER 4

Moving on from the National Service Framework for Mental Health: the social inclusion agenda

BARONESS MOLLY MEACHER and MASON FITZGERALD

An examination of practical – and comparatively simple – methods of psychological support to assist many of those on incapacity benefit with a diagnosed mental illness to return to work – with obvious personal, social and economic benefits. This pioneering approach is to be replicated nationally.

INTRODUCTION

The achievement of the *National Service Framework (NSF) for Mental Health*[1] has been to inject resources into new ways of responding to mental health problems, which better reflect the needs and wishes of service users. This has occurred in both the primary and secondary sectors.

Primary care

About 30% of people who go to a general practitioner (GP) present with mental health problems. Traditionally the response from a GP would be to prescribe medication, although we know that the majority of patients would prefer therapy.[2] For the first time a national initiative to promote psychological therapies in general practice was stimulated by the *National Service Framework*. The *National Health Service (NHS) Plan*[3] then set a target of 1000 primary care workers to be in post by December 2004. This target stimulated the employment of psychology graduates in primary care, albeit with minimal or no training in evidence-based therapies. It was, however, an important start. We discuss the next steps below.

Secondary care

The *National Service Framework* (*NSF*) shifted the focus of psychiatry to a significant degree from a hospital setting to the community. The change has been substantial and generally positive. When the *NSF* was written, the secondary services comprised inpatient beds and community mental health teams (CMHTs). If the generic CMHT could not manage the patient at home, there was little option but to admit the patient to a ward. The NSF presented the case for three new types of specialist community teams, with the following functions:

1   assertive outreach teams – to provide intensive care for people with the most complex social needs, many with a forensic history and difficult to engage with services

2   crisis resolution teams – multi-disciplinary services providing 24-hour specialist assessment and treatment, enabling people in crisis to be cared for in their own homes, where possible, and providing the route into hospital when this is needed

3   early intervention teams – to provide psychological and other services as soon as a young person's psychiatric problems (generally psychoses) come to the attention of doctors or others in a position to refer.

Today a Mental Health Trust can expect to have each of the above teams available to their population. Any patient referred by their GP to the secondary mental health services can expect to have their case reviewed by the assessment team of the local CMHT and, where necessary, referred on to one of the specialist teams.

The system of community teams does, and we believe will increasingly, reduce significantly the need for inpatient admission.[4]

THE SOCIAL INCLUSION AGENDA

The Social Exclusion Unit report of June 2004[5] took us forward from the *NSF* towards the normalisation of life for people with long-term mental health problems. What did this mean in practice? It meant the involvement of this traditionally isolated group in community activities which brought them into contact with others. In the past and, too often, today a person with long-term mental health problems will have no job, no training programme, no other activities and will spend most of their time alone.

TODAY'S AGENDA

This chapter will examine five major initiatives now under way, which will shift the world of the mental health service user sharply away from the isolation of the past:

1 employment and welfare reform
2 the nationwide development of psychological therapies
3 flexible responses to psychotic crises
4 normalisation and integration
5 Foundation Trust status.

EMPLOYMENT AND WELFARE REFORM

It is clear that obtaining employment and remaining in employment can provide many valuable benefits to those who suffer from mental health problems. Apart from the obvious financial independence, employment can support a recovery-based model of treatment by providing a strong sense of self-worth, and enable people to be fully involved in the local community.

The Social Exclusion Unit report set out a 27-point action plan for the development of better access to employment and social, educational and community activity. It aims to improve the availability of vocational advisors to people under mental healthcare and reduce the number of people receiving incapacity benefits on the grounds of mental ill-health.

The report highlighted that only 24% of adults with long-term mental health problems are in work, which is the lowest employment rate for any of the main groups of disabled people. The situation is worse for people with severe mental health problems, with one study showing that only 8% of people were in paid work. Professionals are often felt to have low expectations of what people with mental health problems can achieve. There is a lack of clear responsibility for promoting vocational and social outcomes, and a lack of ongoing support to enable people to work.

A number of Trusts across the country have introduced innovative approaches which are making an impact in this area. In London, the South West London and St George's Mental Health Trust has successful Individual Placement and Support programmes in place, and the Routes 2 Employment programme, a joint NHS Live project in North and East London, is opening up opportunities for open employment in new ways with the support of private employers.

In February 2006 the Department of Health and the Department for Work and Pensions published *Vocational Services for People with Severe Mental Health Problems: commissioning guidance*, through the National Social Inclusion

Programme.[6] The report sets out performance indicators in the commissioning framework for vocational services, and provides that there should be one clinical vocational lead (a mental health professional with an interest in vocational rehabilitation) in each CMHT or specialist team, as well as one employment specialist per clinical team. We would argue that employment specialists should have suitable skills and attributes. People other than mental health professionals may often be the best people for this work. They should manage a vocational caseload of up to 25 people at any one time, and have key links to specialist and mainstream vocational providers, including Jobcentre Plus. Their role is to manage all phases of the vocational service (engagement, assessment, job placement and ongoing support), working for steady progress but at an appropriate pace for the service user they are supporting.

The challenge is now for Mental Health Trusts and Primary Care Trusts (PCTs) to fund and establish clinical vocational leads and employment specialists in teams, and therefore ensure that a vocational service is available to support every service user's path to recovery, so that return to work is seen as the norm and included in care plans from the onset of illness or any subsequent episode. This work is crucial to the success of the social inclusion agenda, as it supports a much-needed paradigm shift, i.e. that those who suffer from poor mental health should be recognised and treated as full members of society, and given appropriate support to enable them to fulfil their potential during all stages of their illness and recovery.

WELFARE REFORM

The Welfare Reform Act 2007 will reduce the number of people dependent upon disability benefits by one million over ten years. Just over half of those affected have a mental health problem as their primary or secondary diagnosis.

The crucial issue for claimants will be whether they are assessed as having a 'limited capability for work' and are thus eligible for the Employment and Support Allowance (ESA). This allowance will replace Incapacity Benefit (IB) and Income Support paid on the basis of incapacity. There will be a 13-week assessment phase for all ESA claimants. During this period people will be paid an 'assessment phase' rate of ESA at the level of the jobseekers' allowance. The rate of the ESA will be above the long-term rate of IB. However, the age-related and dependent additions will no longer be paid. People with more serious disabilities assessed as having 'limited capability for work-related activity' will belong to the 'Support Group' and will receive a higher rate of benefit. The Support Group will not be expected to engage in work-related activity, whereas the work-related activities group will have a work-focused health assessment to establish what the claimant can do and what help they will need to return to work. Based upon that assessment, they will have to attend a series of work-focused interviews on a monthly basis and, in due course, will be required to participate in work-related activities if they are to continue qualifying for full ESA benefit.

For people with fluctuating mental health problems, the new system is potentially alarming. The Pathways for Work pilots, upon which the legislation is based, helped many return to work but failed to significantly help people with mental health problems. The new system will be less well funded, contracted out to private providers, operated on a payment-by-results basis, with no condition-management support. Staff are likely to be less well trained than Pathways staff.

The success of the scheme for people with mental health problems will depend upon a number of significant changes. The NHS will need to provide quality evidence-based psychological therapy for all those affected; also quality employment-support services. Employers will need a new attitude for staff with anxiety, depression or related problems, and the Department for Work and Pensions will need to customise their linking rules to enable people with fluctuating disorders to move in and out of work (on and off benefit) with minimum disruption to their incomes.

An automatic system for the re-establishment of benefit would be a major step forward for those with severe and enduring mental illness. Benefits (including housing benefits) should be automatically restored following confirmation from mental health professionals that the service user is once again unable to work. This policy proposal reflects the reality of the experiences of many service users and would help to provide an equitable and whole systems approach to the problems they face, by encouraging those with severe and enduring mental illness to take advantage of employment opportunities without undue fear of the medium-term financial consequences.

THE NATIONWIDE DEVELOPMENT OF PSYCHOLOGICAL THERAPIES

The expansion of evidence-based psychological therapies will be essential if people with long-term mental health problems, including anxieties and depression, are to be reintroduced to work and a normal life.

Therapies are now available which have been tested in hundreds of clinical trials where sufferers are randomly assigned between therapy and some alternative. We know from the research that some therapies are as effective as drugs in the short run, and in the longer run these therapies have more lasting benefits than drugs.

The therapy most strongly recommended by the National Institute of Clinical Excellence (NICE) is cognitive behavioural therapy (CBT). For example, for panic disorder and generalised anxiety disorder NICE identifies 'the interventions that have evidence for the longest duration of effect, in descending order as a) psychological therapy (cognitive behavioural therapy (CBT); b) pharmacological therapy; and c) self-help using written materials – the use of written materials to help people understand their psychological problems and learn ways to overcome them by changing their behaviour – based on CBT principles'.[7]

For schizophrenia, NICE recommends 'psychological treatment should be an indispensable part of the treatment options available for service users and their families in the effort to promote recoveries'.[8] The report notes that those with the best evidence of effectiveness are cognitive behavioural therapy and family interventions. These should be used to prevent relapse, reduce symptoms, increase insight and promote adherence to medication.[9]

These are revolutionary ideas for improving the treatment of schizophrenia. The duration of CBT is clearly important for this group of patients. NICE argues that treatment of at least ten sessions over at least six months will be necessary to achieve the desired outcomes.

Family interventions should, says NICE, be available to the families of people with schizophrenia who are living with or in close contact with a service user. In particular these interventions should be offered if the service user has recently relapsed, or is considered at risk of relapse, or has persisting symptoms. Again, interventions over more than six months are necessary to achieve the desired results.

The implementation of these recommendations is in its early stages.

NATIONAL PILOTS

The Government has funded two pilots to test the most appropriate model for the delivery of psychological therapies, one in Newham in East London and another in Doncaster, to test the hypothesis that:

1 the provision of stepped improvements in access to evidence-based psycho-therapies for adults of working ages with common mental health problems in the primary and other community settings will improve people's well-being and help them to stay in or return to work, and that

2 these increases in psychological therapies capacity could be largely self-financing by a commensurate reduction in IBs and health service efficiencies.

The Newham Project will deliver evidence-based psychological therapies linked to a voluntary sector employment service to maintain people with mental health problems in work and support people back to work. This project will include assessment for provision of psychological treatment, including individual and group CBT; level one interventions; computerised CBT, self-help material and exercise.

The Doncaster project will deliver high-volume, low-intensity psychological therapies with close involvement from the Chamber of Commerce. This will be linked to an awareness-raising programme for local business which will target 1000 companies; and will support small- and medium-sized businesses to maintain people in employment and assist their return to work.

Professor Lord Richard Layard's proposal is for a high-quality therapy service to which GPs, Occupational Health services and job centre staff could refer people whose lives and work are being wrecked by mental health problems. People should also be able to refer themselves.[10]

Therapists should work in teams which include senior therapists who can supervise the junior therapists, monitor the results of the therapy and provide on-the-job training. The typical team would cover a population of about 200 000 (250 teams nationally). Each team would have a base location of operation but most of the therapy would be delivered at the most convenient place for the client – the GP's surgery, the jobcentre or workplace. The hub-and-spoke model, the team office for supervision, training and support of the service and local service delivery, would ensure high quality and effectiveness.

Professor Lord Layard estimates that it will take seven years to train the necessary 10 000 therapists in evidence-based therapies to deliver the service. Some 5000 of these should be clinical psychologists whose training should be focused more strongly in the direction of evidence-based therapies. The remaining 5000 therapists could be trained from the 60 000 nurses, social workers, occupational therapists and counsellors already working within NHS mental health services.

FLEXIBLE RESPONSES TO PSYCHOTIC CASES

In future, every Mental Health Trust will need a range of services available to deal with psychotic cases if the trauma of detentions in hospital are to be minimised. These services, which together could represent the optimum range of crisis services, are:

1   the crisis resolution team
2   the crisis house

3   the modern day hospital or day therapy centre
4   inpatient admission.

1 The crisis resolution team (also referred to as a home treatment team)
The crisis resolution team is at the heart of crisis work. The aims of the team are to provide a rapid response to a service user in acute crisis, to assess and provide intensive support, monitoring and practical help. Where possible, admission to hospital will be avoided. No admission should take place before the crisis team has done all it can to avoid that eventuality.

The model
The approach of a crisis team is flexible and responsive to the individual crisis. If a service user is suicidal, the team will seek to motivate the individual's social network of family and friends. They may organise for a rota of people to stay with the service user or alternatively for the user to stay with a family member throughout the crisis. In the event of a housing crisis, the team will contact the housing department, or if the electricity has been disconnected the team will organise a re-connection. Nurses monitor medication and ensure compliance. The care plan may include work with families, helping them to understand the illness and behaviours associated with it, or counselling of the service user.

As important as the therapeutic intervention is help with practical problems – benefits, shopping, cooking and signposting to other services.

The time commitment can be considerable. A mental health assessment takes about two hours. Then, depending upon the level of risk, staff will visit up to three times a day for an average of one hour for each visit. The work may continue at this level of intensity for about a week. The care will be reviewed daily and, as the level of risk declines, visits will be reduced to one a day for an average of six weeks, though this could be extended to 12 weeks if necessary. The service user will be passed on to the Community Mental Health Team for ongoing monitoring, and to other services as necessary.

Options for the crisis team
If the crisis cannot be managed at home, the crisis team has a number of options:
➤ referral to the crisis house
➤ referral to the therapeutic day hospital (*see* paragraph below)
➤ seeking admission of the patient to an inpatient ward.

2 The crisis house

From the 1940s alternatives to psychiatric hospitals have been sought. The Henderson Hospital – a therapeutic community – and RD Laing's 'communes' of the 1960s were early examples. We want to focus upon a more recent model inspired by Paul Sherman of the East London and the City Mental Health NHS Trust. The model was created in partnership between the Trust and a voluntary organisation, Heritage Care. This model draws on the experience and ideas of crisis houses across the country.

The crisis house is jointly funded by the Trust and by Supporting People monies from Central Government. Staff include a psychologist who is the therapy lead, counsellors who engage service users in talking therapies, and senior support workers who provide practical help. The quality of the service is monitored by the local authority through an annual quality assessment.

Service users receive an individualised service with a focus on therapy and communication aimed at meeting their needs and helping them to gain insight into their problems. All are treated with dignity and respect. If medication is needed to help recovery, then the service user will be assisted to come to terms with that.

Ideally a person will go to a crisis house *before* they become so unwell that detention is inevitable, and while they still have some insight and are therefore accessible to sensitive communication.

Service users often arrive in a degree of chaos and need structure. The day is organised as far as possible like that of a domestic home, where users participate in the normal jobs of tidying up and cooking, for example. The house needs to be clear about the beginning, middle and end of a user's stay. The initial assessment should be done with the service user and staff who should jointly plan key areas of work and key indicators to determine when progress is made. Clear evidence of progress encourages the individual. By planning the exit strategy from day one, the crisis house is able to achieve an average length of stay of about three weeks.

A doctor from the crisis team visits the crisis house once a week to assess all the users placed there and to monitor their medication. Most residents at the crisis house are a suicide risk but none is detained under the Mental Health Act.

Time spent at the crisis house should be the start of identifying longer-term needs for therapy and support. An important part of this is that users establish their own networks so that they meet on a regular basis and support each other.

3 The modern day hospital or day therapy centre

This facility offers a safe place in a therapeutic environment with a structured programme to meet individual needs identified in a full initial assessment. The programme includes a range of verbal and non-verbal therapies, creative and work-based interventions, and users attend five days per week and for up to three hours at weekends. The programme also seeks to understand and address the families' dynamics and any difficulties they and the service users may be experiencing. The average length of stay is about two months.

Service users will have been assessed as acute and in need of hospital admission if not admitted to the day hospital. The hospital operates a no-waiting list policy. It has 20 places and closes to admissions when it is full.

4 Inpatient admission

When there is no alternative to admission, the community teams will nevertheless be on hand to ensure that the patient spends the shortest possible time in hospital. Early discharge to the crisis team or crisis house will always be considered.

NORMALISATION AND INTEGRATION

Mental health services have so far worked to shift the focus of treatment from medication alone to a more balanced approach, generally involving medication *and* psychological therapies and social interventions. To complement the development of therapies, we are seeing a further shift towards 'normal' activities: open employment; sports like football; joining clubs and libraries; not only art therapy but also art; not only drama therapy but also drama. Both art therapy and drama therapy are powerful therapeutic tools. But if a service user is an artist or a skilled actor, they will manage their condition more effectively and will live a happier and more fulfilled life if they can follow their vocation.

The Core Arts project in Hackney has discovered artists amongst their service users. Their work has been shown at two West End exhibitions and sales are going well for the most talented.

The Mellow Black Drama project has produced plays written and performed in part by service users, not only enhancing the confidence of the individuals but also educating staff and communities about service users' experiences of racism.

In East London, severely unwell schizophrenic young black men are amongst those who have made remarkable strides through their involvement in the Trust football team. The benefits have been many. Players smoke less,

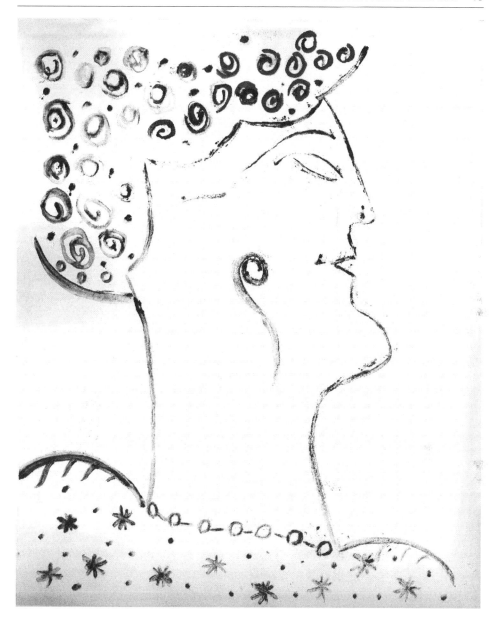

FIGURE 4.1 *Woman's Profile* by Maria de Brito, Core Arts. Reproduced with kind permission.

eat better and have lost weight. Their symptoms have lessened and their motivation to manage their illness has improved dramatically. This project has inspired other Trusts to create football teams. The idea is catching on fast.

More generally, normalisation also means users going to the local community swimming pool, bingo club or library. Segregation is out; integration is now the objective.

FOUNDATION TRUST STATUS

The creation of Foundation Trusts, which are locally accountable through their members and governors, provides an opportunity for a real say in how services are developed and delivered, and also an opportunity and obligation for Foundation Trusts to deliver a comprehensive Patient and Public Involvement strategy, encompassing the wider community and seeking to change the attitudes of employers. Indeed, the NHS Foundation Trust Code of Governance requires Foundation Trusts to make available a public document that sets out its policy on the involvement of members, patients, clients and the local community at large.

There are currently 51 Foundation Trusts, and many more NHS Trusts are on the same path. One part of the application process is the requirement to conduct an intensive, 12-week public consultation. These consultations are used to reach out to groups that previously have not had sufficient involvement in mental health services, including a large number of black and ethnic minority community groups where appropriate. The consultation exercise is also used as an opportunity to raise awareness and understanding of mental health issues. Local community fairs and public events raise the profile of mental health issues and services in the community and attempt to challenge the stigma of mental health.

Every Foundation Trust has a Board of Governors, which is made up of elected members of the public, as well as staff, and appointed governors from local Primary Care Trusts PCTs, (LAs), universities, and voluntary organisations. The role of a Board of Governors is to represent the interests of the Trust's members and partner organisations in the local health economy in the governance of the Trust, and to regularly feed back information about the Trust, its vision and performance to the constituencies and stakeholder organisations that either elected or appointed them. The governors must be consulted by the Board of Directors in the forward planning of the Trust.

The creation of Foundation Trusts signifies a fundamental shift in the balance of power in the NHS, devolving accountability from Whitehall to local communities, and offers an opportunity to promote the social inclusion agenda. It also provides actual and aspiring Foundation Trusts with an opportunity and obligation to devise and deliver a comprehensive Public and Patient Involvement strategy that takes account of service users, carers and the wider community at all levels, therefore ensuring that local people have a real influence in the shaping and delivery of their own mental health services.

CONCLUSION

The 1950s saw a revolution in mental health services following the introduction of psychotropic drugs. These enabled much shorter hospital stays and the closure of the isolated asylums of a by-gone age. The first quarter of the 21st century will witness an equally dramatic change from an isolated life in hospitals, hostels, group homes and day centres to one of integration: more open employment, use of local facilities, more integrated housing, and much less use of detention in hospital as evidence-based psychological therapies enable people to manage their conditions at home most of the time. This chapter set out some of the steps we all need to take to turn aspiration into actuality.

REFERENCES

 1 Department of Health. *National Service Framework for Mental Health: Modern Standards and Service Models.* London: Department of Health; 1999.
 2 Chilver C, Dewey M, Fielding K *et al.* Anti-depressant drugs and generic counselling for treatment of major depression in primary care. *BMJ.* 2001; **322**: 2.
 3 Department of Health. *The NHS Plan: a plan for investment, a plan for reform.* London: Department of Health; 2000.
 4 Glover G, Arts G, Babu KS. Crisis resolution/home treatment teams and psychiatric admission rates in England. *Br J Psychiatry.* 2006; **189**: 441–5.
 5 Social Exclusion Unit. *Mental Health and Social Exclusion.* London: ODPM; 2004.
 6 Department of Health, Department for Work and Pensions. *Vocational Services for People with Severe Mental Health Problems: commissioning guidance.* London: Department of Health; 2006.
 7 National Institute for Clinical Excellence. *Anxiety: management of anxiety in adults in primary, secondary and community care.* London: National Institute for Clinical Excellence; 2004.
 8 Ibid.
 9 National Institute for Clinical Excellence. *Schizophrenia Core Interventions in the Treatment and Management of Schizophrenia in Primary and Secondary Care.* London: National Institute for Clinical Excellence; 2002.
10 Layard R. *The Depression Report.* London: London School of Economics, the Centre for Economic Performance; 2006.

CHAPTER 5

A GP's view: interview with Dr Helen Pelendrides

Dr Helen Pelendrides spent 15 years working as a GP in a large, multi-site practice in North London serving about 11 000 patients, before moving to a smaller practice where she currently works with some 3500 patients in a more deprived catchment area. Her experience working in two London boroughs with dissimilar provision for mental healthcare gives her considerable insight into metropolitan realities in treatment terms. The interview took place with Charles Kaye in December 2006.

'It is an exciting time to be a GP, with unprecedented opportunities to improve patient care, but improving morale is a complex issue and there is no simple solution. Excessive workloads are a major cause of stress, but two things could make a big difference. First, to take every possible step to strengthen the doctor–patient relationship. Increasingly we are dealing with patients with complex problems who deserve more consultation time and doctors and patients know that ten minutes is insufficient. Efforts to increase the average consultation time are therefore to be welcomed. The second is to improve the support for GPs to deliver patient care – such as being able to order more X-rays and scans and having more responsive hospital services . . . Life without general practitioners is not possible and it is about time we stood up for the thousands of GPs who are making a real difference to patients' lives up and down the country on a daily basis.'

Letter to *The Times*, 8 January 2007, from Professor Mayur Lakhani, Chairman, Royal College of General Practitioners.
Reproduced with permission.

THE PRACTICE

HP I have had the good fortune to work in different environments and I think that is quite useful because mental health and the care of mental health very much depends on postcode.

Currently, I work in a suburb in Wood Green in North London, which is in Haringey, a much more deprived part of London than Barnet where I worked before. It's a much smaller practice, 3500 patients. They are mainly of the same ethnic background because, traditionally, the practice has been Greek speaking, started off by my father who was the first Greek-speaking doctor in the area. A largely Greek Cypriot population who tended to come to a doctor who could speak to them in their native tongue. So the tradition is that we have got very much a Greek Cypriot community plus people who have moved into the area more recently. So the mixture has increased recently with a large Eastern European influx.

We have a large proportion of new patients, mainly young Bulgarians, but with some Poles. They come with their own problems, obviously in a completely different environment with language problems, with economic and financial problems, social problems. We are now starting to have to face an entirely new area of health concerns. This is a small practice, suburban with a different mental health set-up from Barnet where I worked for 15 years in a much larger practice, 11 500 patients and six partners. The set-up in Barnet was organised in a totally different way and with a very multi-ethnic population even though it is a nice affluent suburb. The population mix was much greater than where I am now.

PATIENTS AND MENTAL ILLNESS

HP It is a major feature of our work whether it is minor mental health or major mental health. It is something which we see, if not on daily basis, certainly three or four times a week and I just looked at my population figures before I came, to give myself an idea. On the serious mental health register, we have 50 patients, which is 1.4% of our population, and on the current depression register, we have got 137, which is roughly 4%. With regard to dementia, we only have 11 because we don't look after any homes so it's very low. There are no residential or nursing homes, so these are people who are still looked after within their normal environment and haven't moved into care. That's only 0.3% of our population, which I think is low compared to other neighbouring practices which look after a home where there would be a lot of elderly mental health problems. So, that's our current population mix. I think treating mental illness is core to general practice. I don't think anybody can separate the two and it comes into consultations in all sorts of different ways, as I'm sure you know. And it's up to us to tease out where the problems actually lie.

We recently had a refugee doctor with us: it's very interesting to show someone who is from a different culture completely, who has never been taught why patients present to the doctor, because in her background people went to the specialist of their choice. Therefore, if they went to a physician, they believed that there was something wrong with their heart and if they went to dermatologist, they had decided their problem was in the skin. Here we are seeing people presenting with one thing who actually have got something completely different going on in the background and we have to work out what the right agenda is. To explain that to someone who really hasn't seen medical problems in that way is very interesting.

Very few patients will come and say 'I feel really low'. Some will, but the majority won't and they will come with something else and just looking at them and hearing the story, you think, 'this doesn't fit, this is not really the major problem here' and then you have to tease it out. I think experience is probably the most important thing. As time goes on, you get better at picking up when there is a problem and when not to take things at face value. I think that the training we were given in general practice gave us a lot of help in looking for this kind of problem and, although at the beginning you are floundering with all the different things that are going on, as time goes on, I think you can start to sieve out and find the psychological aspects of things.

CK So, would she not have seen much mental illness?

HP I don't think she had seen any mental illness. Her experience was quite limited. She had come from Romania and she was debating whether general practice was the right way forward or the hospital, so this was a taster of general practice for four weeks and after a patient had left, I said to her, 'Well, what do you think they came for today? It wasn't the cough, I can't remember what the minor symptom was but that was not the reason, was it?' And she said, 'Well actually, it's funny you should say that, I thought it was a bit odd'. But, you know, to her the idea that the patient has to have a ticket to come to the doctor and actually behind that ticket, there is something that could well be a mental/psychological problem was quite new to her.

CK Does that mean your training offered you something that her training hasn't, then?

HP I most definitely think that.

With our three-year general practice rotation within hospital plus the one-year within practice, I think that it is very well drawn out that you have to question what is the patient's agenda. Why are they here? Why have they come today? What was a chronic problem that became acute today? And often it is a psychological reason. It is not because the physical symptoms have suddenly got worse. There is some other reason which has made their coping mechanism crash on that day. Looking at it from her perspective was really interesting for me, I must say.

CK Is the way that you practise different in the smaller practice where you are now from what it was like in the much larger one? Do you have a different relationship with the patients?

HP Yes, I think it is. The main reason is because I know most of the patients, I can't say I know them all, but I know a great many of them and the ones who I see, I tend to know more about because it has built up. Although I was in the other practice for longer, I can't say that I knew the patients in the same way because of the numbers and they would move around the practice.

WORKING WITH THE MENTAL HEALTH SERVICES

CK And what about the relationship with the PCT [Primary Care Trust] services and the multifarious teams that are everywhere?

HP Yes, the problem for us is that communication with a member of a team who has seen a patient is very difficult, and they asked us this question recently when they were setting up the library service. There was a questionnaire about what we find is difficult and what works well. Communicating with a member of the team is almost impossible, because how it works in Haringey is that the community mental health team have a duty officer and they prefer you not to ring up because they prefer not to answer the phone, so referrals get posted or faxed through to them and they have meetings and they prioritise and decide who does what. But if a patient has been seen by a member of that team, actually speaking to them in order to get some kind of follow-up or to find out what's happened or when they are going to be seen again if the patient hasn't understood – any kind of communication with an individual – is almost impossible.

CK So your contact with these services, which presumably are going to pick up all your serious situations, is actually quite difficult.

HP It's not ideal. I think getting the initial information from us to them is fine, because if it is faxed or posted, it gets to them. They know what they are going to do but I don't. I don't know when the patient is going to be seen, so if I am worried about someone, I have got no idea when they are going to be seen. I usually rely on the patient to tell me as that is easier than finding out what they [the community mental health team] intend to do. Once the patient has been seen, that's fine because usually there is continuity from week to week and they will be seen for a series of sessions. Then once they have been discharged, it gets a bit tricky again, usually a summary will follow with a plan of what has happened and medication change and follow-up, what they have told the patient to do if there is a crisis, usually that will follow; sometimes it doesn't and sometimes it is in limbo, not knowing quite who is going where and who is going to pick up the next bit, whilst we are waiting for something else to happen. So, it's not ideal.

CK As far as you can judge, how effective is all this with the patients?

HP I'm not sure what each team is supposed to do but, from what I have understood so far, and it may not be completely correct, is that there is a sort of general community mental health team. There is also a sub-section of that which is more minor – hand-holding GP-type problems for which they hope they will be able to offer six to eight sessions of counselling – but it's not working terribly well at the moment. They haven't got enough manpower but they are thinking along those lines and probably we are going to be able to refer straight into that stream without having to go through the main block, but it's not entirely clear and it is new. And then there is the very severe – psychotherapy, long-term counselling, personality disorders, transsexual – stuff, all of that which is really going to be years, which goes a different way but often we may not realise that is what is going to happen. And within their own team, within the Community Mental Health, the umbrella organisation, I have only recently realised there is a refugee service which I didn't even know about. You know, I have been working here three years and I didn't know about this until a referral came back and they said, 'This should really go back to the Refugee Clinic because that is the best place'. Well, I agree entirely, if only I'd known.

And again, that's postcode dependent so if it is the wrong area and we are right on the verge, we are on the border between one PCT and another. So our patients are on both sides.

CK So some will have a refugee clinic and some won't?

HP That's right and we have to remember which is which and how to refer them. There is a psychiatrist as part of the team, but not a direct patient-with-psychiatrist clinic appointment – that is a separate issue. So all of this goes on as part of a community team. I think the psychiatrist sits in on their assessment meetings and the triage and the prioritising.

CK Yet you are supposed to be an expert on this because the patient comes to you, 'Oh well, the doctor will know what's what!'

HP I know the initial entry point but quite what happens after that is quite mysterious to me.

CK So people from the various community mental health teams, would they ever come to the surgery for any reason? Would you ever see them?

HP No. I think probably because we are a small practice. If we were a larger practice and referred a large number, I think they might actually consider seeing patients within our premises because of the workload.

CK And are you atypical in being a small practice?

HP No, in Haringey it's not atypical at all.

CK So what if you have got a serious crisis on your hands?

HP There is an 'urgent care referral pathway'. The jargon's good. So what that means is they will respond within the next day or two – *working* day or two. Anyway, the early intervention team would usually see the patient at home. If they think staying at home is safe and they can continue with input from them, the patient is safe there, then they will carry on visiting probably daily for a period of time until some other plan would take over. If she or he is very unstable, they will admit from there or give instructions to the emergency reception at St Anne's that the patient is to be given permission to turn up at any time and to be reassessed. So that's the short term. If, another long list, they can't cope at home but don't need to be in hospital – they can't cope because there is no food, there's nobody to go out shopping, there's no electricity, they haven't paid the electricity bill so it has been cut off; whatever, the crisis is in the environment at home – then there is a crisis hostel in Hornsey where patients can be admitted by the mental health team where all this is provided – so food and light and heat and everything else is provided.

CK Then as their GP, what do you know? As these things develop?

HP As these things develop, there is usually a fax from one of these points, even from the crisis team going to visit and what's happened, or they have been admitted to the hostel or they have been admitted to hospital.

If they have been admitted to hospital, we hear nothing for weeks, sometimes months, until a phone call comes through saying, 'Will you come and do this section form?' or they get discharged and a discharge summary comes through. So, I think we do hear about what's happening at different steps of the way through the fax, which is very useful because otherwise it would come through the post, it would all be over by the time we found out what was happening. So yes, that's good, I have to say, yes, that communication is useful.

CK Do you regard that as a good service or are there ways in which you would like to see it change?

HP When things reach crisis point, I think it works well.

CK Do you think the patients understand the rhythm of the service or is it somewhat disjointed?

HP I don't think so, no. I think the patients are confused. They are already confused because that is why they are in that situation. I don't think they understand how it works and how can they? If I don't understand it after three years, how can they possibly understand it? So I think at that point, they are relieved that somebody is taking an interest in their problem.

I think we have to be able to work the system and that is our responsibility to the patient, and if we can't do it and get it right – get the patient to the right point of help – then we are failing them. I am sure I have done that and I haven't got to the right place at the right time when I should have done, so that makes me feel uncomfortable. The people who were not acutely ill are the ones that miss out and that makes me uncomfortable, as well as we have nothing to plug the gap.

So the ones in crisis get sorted fairly well, the ones with the severe mental health get picked up and get sorted in one way or another, but the ones with the unhappy families and the lingering problems of childhood sexual abuse and now needing to face it, or the unpleasant husband or the bullying at work, those people are the ones that we don't help very well.

CHOICE

CK   In the context of mental illness, what do you think 'choice' means for your patients?

HP   They have choice in as far as who they see in general practice, so they can choose which doctor to see. They can choose to go to another practice if they feel we are unhelpful or our approach is not friendly: that is a real choice. But what happens in secondary care is there is no choice available. There is no choice because it is all postcode led, the services are based not on the GP surgery but where a patient lives.

Because historically, the geographical bond is between Social Services and Health and had to be more or less what they call 'co-terminous'. Over time, everything has built up within a particular area so the consultants are paid by Haringey PCT to see Haringey residents. So, if one of my patients is over the border in Enfield, then that immediately eliminates any of this choice of care and it means they have to go to an Enfield set-up which is organised in a different way, paid for in a different way. There is no choice.

There may be choice once they have been seen for the first assessment – if they particularly dislike the person they have to deal with, they may ask to see someone else but within the same set-up. And they certainly can't go to another hospital. Psychiatric services are based at that – that's why our patients don't like St Anne's; they can't go anywhere else because that's the only site with inpatient beds they can access if they need to be admitted.

Well, I think mental health is a monopoly situation, isn't it? It is a monopoly and it's always been geographical and postcode related, so a patient who lives in Haringey can't see a psychiatrist in Enfield because the funding will not allow since that is the structure of the psychiatric service. There is no choice.

CK   Is there choice for the GP?

HP   Yes. When we are referring people for other problems, physical problems, we often will choose who the right person might be. I mean, the patient is given a choice and if they don't want to go there, then fine, they will go wherever they want to go within limits, but we often know who the right person is to send them to because of his particular interest, particular skills and expertise. We don't have a choice in which psychiatrist to treat our patients. There is one allocated to a subset of postcodes. So in Haringey, the area is patched up four ways, I think; for our area, we only have one psychiatrist.

CK Do you ever meet the consultant psychiatrist? Do you ever have contact?

HP I met the one that has now gone when I went to sign a section form. I haven't met the new one. He has been in post probably close to a year now.

Well in our area, we have no choice; we can only use that one consultant psychiatrist out of the team. I am not sure how many there are now. Even a patient who had a long-standing relationship with one particular psychiatrist was not allowed to continue to see that individual because of the restructuring of the area, and that's it. What happened with that patient was interesting. He was a chronic schizophrenic and he was really burnt out, so he didn't really need very much. But losing that relationship with the psychiatrist, who he felt had offered him a great deal over the years, was so important to him that he was prepared to leave the practice – us – where he had been registered for 30 years and go to another practice and register there, leaving the rest of his family with us, because that particular psychiatrist did a session in that building and, if he was registered there, he would be entitled to go to that clinic. It must have been a very difficult decision for him to make, and all credit to him for doing it. I think it took real guts for him to do that, and that's fine, but he was prepared to do that in order to exercise what choice he had.

CK So that's a classic example of the system forcing behaviour on the individual rather than the other way around.

HP Yes, although this was an exceptional situation.

CK But choice in psychiatric care is much more limited than in acute care?

HP Yes, because our relationship doesn't matter all, because we are not going to choose someone who is particularly empathic with that problem because there is no choice.

TALKING THERAPIES

HP Certainly in Haringey, talking therapies are the biggest problem from the GP perspective because there is a huge waiting list. The assessment process has to be jumped through by every patient before they can access talking therapy. The wait is off-putting. I mean, if I was in that situation, I wouldn't want to wait a year to be able to talk to someone.

CK   Can the wait be that long?

HP   It can be a year. The more in-depth psychological support is 18 months.

CK   Does that mean that it's largely ineffective?

HP   Some of them will benefit but by the time they reach that stage– they have also gone through some consideration in their own minds. Maybe they have had help from the mental health charities, maybe they have helped themselves. I try to encourage people to do self-help and use CBT [cognitive behavioural therapy] on the internet, 'beating the blues' and accessing other help whilst they are waiting. Not everybody has the resources to do that – the language, the internet access, the capacity, the motivation. So it's all very well saying, 'You go and do this', but they may not have the necessary resources to do it. Just recently, Haringey have actually tried to make things a little bit easier. There is now a walk-in, a drop-in centre at the Library from the end of last month, with access to a counsellor. It can be a self-referral or from a health professional of any kind.

   I think there is a movement afoot to try and buy some of the internet programs and have them in some facility within Haringey so that people can perhaps access them – again, in the Library. If they are going in to read their newspaper or to use something in the Library, they might actually sit at the computer and use a CBT program.

CK   Do you think that's an effective substitute?

HP   Well, I think it is. Again, if the patient is the right one for that mode of treatment, and it won't suit everyone by any means.

STIGMA

CK   Do you find stigma a real problem in practice?

HP   Yes, it is. I mean, with my populations it is a big problem. Because Cypriots don't like talking about depression, they don't like talking about mental illness. It's all considered madness – any mental health problem is madness – and therefore, although it is the 21st century, there is still a lot of that hanging on, and I have talked to Asian colleagues and I think the same thing applies within their community as well. So, a Greek patient will very rarely come and say they are feeling low and tearful but they will tell you about the headaches and tiredness.

CK That's an additional barrier, yes?

HP Well fortunately, I can understand the culture that they come from so I can usually interpret what's going on and, when you finally crack it and they allow you to get close enough to say, 'Well, do you think you could be depressed?', the relief is huge because, of course, they have been hiding behind all these physical symptoms from their own families, their neighbours and everybody, including me. Because the stigma of mental health problems is so enormous, to finally be able to say, 'Yes, actually that is what's happening, thank God somebody has actually asked me'.

CK But what about serious mental illness in that sort of context?

HP The family skirt around it and it is talked about as 'she's weak and vulnerable, frail' and all sorts of avoidance.

It's avoiding the whole topic of mental health, as if I don't know what really is going on; it's really strange. I've got a computer screen in front of me telling me every single section and admission that happens to their relative and yet they are still talking about how fragile she is, but you have to play ball because that's the only way you can engage with the family. Sometimes the patient will actually be very blunt about the whole situation and not be interested in playing these games at all, but the families will. And so you have got to deal with both sides. And using terms like 'schizophrenia' and 'bipolar affective disorder', I mean that really is very tricky, and understanding and accepting it is a huge problem, yes. So that hasn't gone.

CK Do you think, as far as you can judge, that the psychiatric service is sensitive to these sorts of problems?

HP I don't think so. I think they are much more blunt about it, that's my impression.

CK So they are probably not differentiating a whole lot?

HP I don't think so, and because they are all about transparency and everything being out in the open, I think they want to ignore the stigma aspect of it completely and they want everything to be discussed, which is not necessarily what the family welcome. So they go for the open approach which may actually clash with what everybody else thinks, but I think that's how their training is.

LANGUAGE AND COMMUNICATION

CK   And what about language – is language ever a problem?

HP   Oh, language is a big problem. Because . . . that is one aspect of the counselling service and talking therapies which would be a big problem because we would have to accommodate our patients in their language, because counselling in a foreign language is very difficult.

And I think there is a little bit – the charities have organised some small degree of counselling in Turkish, which is a big language in Haringey, not just Greek. There are some services but they are very small and certainly stretched to accommodate everybody who needs them.

CK   So if you have a patient who comes along and has got this sort of low-grade depression and what would be helpful is counselling, if he or she doesn't have reasonably fluent English . . .

HP   What's the point? Because we had a whole influx of Kosovans several years ago and they did present huge mental health problems. Some genuine post-traumatic stress disorder and some less genuine. The psychiatrists, I think, realised they couldn't unpick what was real and what wasn't because everybody wanted to claim refugee status. So of course, the stories were, though profoundly disturbing, not all of them true. So they actually employed somebody who spoke Albanian for a period of time in order to try and understand the cultural background and the differences between the ethnic Kosovans and the ethnic Albanians and some Bosnians. That was, I imagine, pretty expensive but it was a great service for the Kosovans. A lot of them have been sent back now so we haven't got a problem any more.

CK   And the Bulgarians are another group altogether?

HP   At the moment, the Bulgarian situation is that they are working so hard to earn money to send back home, they haven't got time to be ill, which will have repercussions later on because they can't carry on indefinitely and sending every penny back. So we see them when they are at breakdown but the mental health problems that we were used to with other groups, we haven't dealt with yet.

CK   But presumably, they will be coming along, won't they? There will be crises, yes?

HP   That's right and also the other horrific part of it is that they have . . . if they are not at home and they are working all the time, they can't look after their children. So if they have a baby, the child gets sent back to Bulgaria to be looked after by grandparents and other family, or if it is an older child, it goes back to school in Bulgaria because mum and dad are working.

CK So you are going to get all that family upset later on?

HP Yes, a real upset later on. I don't know whether they are hoping they will be able to save enough in a couple of years and then go back and live more comfortably, but you know . . . Whether that is really going to happen, I don't know. It's a worry for the future.

DUAL DIAGNOSIS

HP There is a service, again it's entirely Haringey or entirely Enfield. It's called BDAS – Barnet Drug and Alcohol Service. It's called DASH in Haringey – Drug and Alcohol Service Haringey – and EGDAS in Enfield. I've got a patient who was being seen by DASH and they had the temerity to move to Enfield and had to start all over again because it was a different service.

CK So you couldn't even continue, even if you were in treatment?

HP Well, he . . . Well, we kept him going until he was seeing EGDAS. We do shared care, so we prescribe Methadone. We do screening and all the rest of it but completely different protocols, completely different pathways for the two neighbouring boroughs, and that's how it goes. It's not good, not enough money. I think patients say that it is a drop-in centre so they spend the whole morning waiting to be seen. But it does exist and I think we are grateful it's there.

CK Is it really 'shared care'?

HP I think my colleague, who does the majority of it, gets a bit fed up because he thinks it's not an equitable share. But I think patients prefer to come to us than to go there. They know they will be seen faster. Some of them have got a relationship with us from before, apart from the drug and alcohol aspect. Some don't but some come just because of that.

CK And presumably, they probably find it less stigmatising, too?

HP I think so.

CK A drop-in centre is not private.

HP That's right and everybody knows why you are there. Whereas at the surgery, you are just sitting with other people who are waiting and you could be anaemic.

CK So that is one part of the service where there is some 'share' in the 'care' as it goes along.

HP   Yes, that's how it is supposed to work. We are supposed to alternate so they come to us and go to the clinic. I am not sure the communication is great. I think we generally rely on the patient, who may not be the best person to tell us what's going on.

IN CONCLUSION

HP   The reality at the moment is that, until we can make up the PCTs' financial deficit, we are not going to do anything different. All we can do is restrict and reduce. We have been told that very clearly. Our PCT Chief Exec is a very hard-nosed individual and she has already told us that we are the highest paid GPs in Europe and, therefore, how dare we moan and whinge. And how dare we not take on lots of extra work and get paid less because, you know, we are already overpaid and her job is on the line, of course.

But we have to be pragmatic and with experience comes realisation that you have got to deal with what you have got and that's it. It could be worse – it could be a different situation where there is no crisis service and that happens.

There are parts of London where there is no extra help and I read somewhere Haringey actually invests more of their budget into mental health than a lot of other PCTs in London, so actually we are blessed.

Yes, so why am I moaning? Of course, it could be better, everything could be better but it's not going to change a lot and unless . . . I don't know, if the Trust was suddenly taken over by private providers, something horrific happened, you know, the mental health in Haringey, the Mental Health Trust was wiped out and a private provider came in, what would they do? They are a 'for profit' company, what would they do differently?

CK   Disappointments?

HP   Well, I think having to send people away before they have had their full time allocation – what *they* would consider to be the right amount of time allocation, because *you* can't ignore the fact that other people are waiting and they have an equal right to your time. So that is unsatisfactory because you may be getting someone you know that, if you had a 50-minute appointment like a counsellor, the outcome would be much better at this point, maybe not longer term but now, you would have made more of an impact. But on the other hand, you owe a duty of care and time-keeping to everybody else, so there is a constant balance going on. I think knowing that there isn't anybody who can carry it on immediately, that is really a frustration because I wouldn't need to spend another half-hour if I could refer that person to a colleague next week and know that they would get picked up at the right time.

COMMENTARY BY THE EDITORS

This conversation is, of course, a snapshot but as such it does offer a glimpse into some of the complexities of mental healthcare in a metropolitan setting. The links and interaction between primary care and the mental health specialist services are certainly not straightforward.

A number of key issues emerge – seen obviously from the point of view of a GP trying to achieve the best for her patients:

➤ awareness of 'ethnic minorities' (and that term has wider dimensions than are usually recognised)
➤ the barriers between the different parts of the healthcare system – where different catchment areas have separate frontiers and very limited interchange, e.g. the 'postcode lottery'
➤ the minimal range of choice available to patients – perhaps restricted in practice to changing their GP
➤ the limited and formalised contact between GP and mental health team(s) – particularly in comparison with the 'acute' health services
➤ the role of the patient as 'go-between', filling the communication gaps
➤ the complexity and apparent inflexibility of service arrangements
➤ the mounting financial pressures being experienced by the PCT which are, of course, passed onto GPs and others
➤ recognition of the value of CBT and efforts to increase access to it
➤ the ever-present shadow of stigma.

CHAPTER 6

Dual diagnosis

LORD VICTOR ADEBOWALE and CAROLINE HAWKINGS

'Holistic' care sometimes sounds like a hollow cliché but the problems of patients with concurrent illnesses bring to the fore the need to have an individual-based service approach which can use specialist services creatively: the service should fit the patient.

BEHIND THE DIAGNOSIS: TREATING INDIVIDUALS

The challenge of 'dual diagnosis' reaches to the heart of what we mean by the term 'holistic care'. It is all too easy to assign a label to an individual who may have complex needs and then deconstruct their challenges according to a clinical diagnosis. This reduces an individual to a convenient category rather than addressing the full complexity of their needs.

Our ultimate goal in social care is to create holistic and wrap-around care that is sufficiently sophisticated to cope with the range of social challenges an individual may experience as a result of mental health, substance misuse and other needs.

'Dual diagnosis' is a potentially unhelpful label, both for the individuals concerned and for the people working with them. It is not a clinical diagnosis and does not indicate a new condition, but only identifies that a person has concurrent needs.

This begs the question: which needs? 'Dual diagnosis' means different things to different professionals. In the learning disability field, it means the co-existence of a mental health problem alongside a learning disability, but the focus of this chapter will be on the co-existence of mental health and substance use problems. Even within this spectrum, the combinations, levels of severity and patterns of substance use or mental illness are as diverse as the individuals themselves. Responses to a person with schizophrenia, who uses heroin, will be different from responses to another who has bipolar disorder and uses cannabis and alcohol. People may also have physical health problems and face social challenges such as poor or non-existent housing, unemployment and isolation. In short, an individual's needs 'are often multiple rather than dual and include social as well as medical needs'.[1]

This is why Department of Health guidance has rightly highlighted the importance of having a locally agreed definition among a range of agencies, but it also explains why in some services achieving a definition has proved so elusive.

Acknowledging the problems associated with it, at times, we shall use the words 'dual diagnosis', but as a shorthand for a much more complex term.

If there is little consensus about what is meant by 'dual diagnosis', there is widespread agreement about the scale of the problem. In the United Kingdom, it is estimated that approximately one-third of psychiatric patients with severe mental illness have a substance misuse problem. In drug and alcohol services, approximately half of clients have some form of mental health problem (most commonly depression or personality disorder).[2]

Research suggests that between 22% and 44% of adult psychiatric patients also have problematic drug or alcohol use, with up to half being drug dependent.[3]

Prevalence among the prison population is high – for example, 79% of male remand prisoners who were drug dependent had two additional mental health disorders.[4]

However, these statistics are likely to be a gross underestimate, since people are usually only given a formal diagnosis if they have severe mental health problems (generally psychotic disorders) and severe substance use problems. Undoubtedly, people with a dual diagnosis are more complex and are often described as being more chaotic, but in today's environment of tightly rationed services, we have to question whether their lives have become more chaotic because the more straightforward lower-level interventions were not available or because services were not able to coordinate support at the time when they needed them.

PROBLEMS WITH THE CURRENT SITUATION

Traditionally, substance misuse services and mental health services have been planned, funded and commissioned separately. This fuels a preoccupation amongst many professionals about what came first – whether a person's substance misuse is primary or secondary to their mental health problem or vice versa. While in some cases, this may be clear, it can be very difficult to distinguish. There is a danger that answering this question and therefore deciding which service should take the lead, may become the focus of assessment instead of a client's needs.

People with dual or complex needs are falling through the gaps – they may have a range of needs, but no 'single' condition which is severe enough to meet the criteria for specialist support. They are therefore presenting at GPs, Accident and Emergency Departments (A&E) and other community services at crisis point. For example, it is not uncommon for people to complete a detoxification for their alcohol problems several times, only to relapse because they cannot access appropriate help for their underlying mental health needs. This is a failure for both practitioners and individuals, who feel discouraged yet again.

Specialist services are rare and frontline staff feel ill-equipped to deal with the range of challenges presented to them. From the outset, the label of dual diagnosis signals that a person has at least two problems, prompting a reaction that a person will be 'double the trouble' and therefore more costly in terms of time and treatment interventions, even before a more detailed assessment and subsequent treatment may begin. There may be diverse and complex needs to be addressed, but an individual should not be 'blamed' for their situation. Furthermore, if a person does not receive appropriate help at the right time, the costs will be far greater, both directly for the individual and the services concerned and indirectly for society at large.

With mental health services already stretched, people with co-existing mental health and substance misuse problems are often neglected. Responses from services vary, and some practitioners are doing excellent work with limited resources. However, more commonly, people are not receiving the services they need and, if they are, they are often discharged too early without adequate care plans or ongoing support. Typically, people have several co-existing problems and wider social care needs, including employment and housing. To quote the King's Fund report *London's State of Mind* (2003), 'Although the complexity of need has increased generally, providers of supported housing are reluctant to accept the most complex and difficult clients'.

It is also easy to forget that people with a dual diagnosis fulfil important roles in the community. As one service user, Lucy, explains, 'When I first entered the mental health system and asked for help, statutory services took my daughter away, which just exacerbated my problems . . . She had been my sole reason for "holding things together". There is already a stigma attached to dual diagnosis, but add to this a mother who has had her child taken away from her because of it, and I felt even more isolated.' With support, Lucy has gradually built up contact and her daughter now stays regularly. An individual must be seen in the wider context of their family and friends. Too often, it is easy to forget that many patients or service users are also parents, employees or carers and should be given support to enable them to continue in those roles.

DUAL DIAGNOSIS: THE POLICY CONTEXT

Despite these problems, the profile of dual diagnosis in the policy agenda has until recently been relatively low. Many policy drivers such as Models of Care or the Updated Drugs Strategy have focused on their core business, offering little guidance about the treatment and support of people who need both mental health and substance misuse services. Even the *National Service Framework for Mental Health* (1999) contained little specific direction about dual diagnosis.

It was not until 2002 that the Department of Health issued the *Policy Implementation Guidance on Dual Diagnosis Good Practice*. It focuses on mainstreaming the care of people with severe mental health problems and problematic substance use, through mental health services taking the primary responsibility for their treatment. Substance misuse agencies (both alcohol and drugs) should provide specialist support, consultancy and training to mental health teams and, where clients have less severe mental health problems, mental health services should provide similar support to substance misuse agencies. It stresses the importance of clear pathways of joint working and treatment, with local implementation teams (LITs) and drug and alcohol action teams taking the lead.

However, the *Review of the Mental Health National Service Framework Five Years On* (2004) found that: only 17% of LITs have a dual diagnosis strategy; planning and commissioning is often poor; many staff in assertive outreach teams have no training in substance misuse, and the evidence base into effective interventions is lacking. In the light of these appalling statistics, the review sets dual diagnosis as one of the priority areas for specialist mental health services and recognises that a 'broad co-ordinated approach' is required. It makes a series of recommendations about the key role of assertive outreach teams and dedicated services for dual diagnosis, improved collaboration between community drug and alcohol teams and mental health teams, better training for mental health staff in the assessment and clinical management of substance misuse, as well as practical steps to prevent drug misuse in inpatient units and cannabis use in people with severe mental illness.

Dual diagnosis was the focus of the *Themed Review* in the assessment of LITs (2006–07), with the aim of identifying 'key issues in relation to the provision of care for individuals with substance use and mental illness'.[5] It will yield valuable qualitative and quantitative information about current service provision. The key question is how the information is used and applied to improve and increase services on the front line.

In spite of these frameworks setting out laudable theory, the reality is very different – as borne out of our experience in the social care organisation Turning Point. In 2008 Turning Point provided some 250 services across a range of settings for people whose lives are affected by mental health issues, substance misuse or a learning disability. We have particular expertise in working with people who have complex needs and are facing multiple social challenges. A large number of our service users have overlapping substance misuse, mental health and other needs and we estimate that at least one in five of people we support with mental health issues also needs help with serious substance misuse.

Having outlined some of the problems and analysis of the current situation, we would now like to turn to some solutions for future service provision. These are informed both by our personal perspectives and the views of people using Turning Point's services.

All the evidence suggests that substance use is usual rather than exceptional for people with mental health issues. Therefore, a mental health service isn't fit for purpose until it has a better understanding and consequently a better response to the needs of people with dual diagnosis. We are the first to acknowledge that dual diagnosis is a challenging area of practice and is associated with poorer treatment outcomes and heavier and more frequent use of services. Solutions need to be tailored to local circumstances and even more so to individuals. We are also aware that provision spans a range of settings and service models operating with vastly different resources. This includes acute inpatient wards and special hospitals, to assertive outreach teams or consultants, GPs, housing agencies – and spans dedicated teams as well as sole dual-diagnosis link workers covering a huge geographical area.

However, we would like to sketch out some broad themes that will help us work towards services that are fit for purpose for the 21st century. We shall consider four areas:

➤ strategic planning
➤ workforce, training and professional roles
➤ provision for black and minority ethnic communities
➤ service delivery.

STRATEGIC PLANNING

Flexible, innovative commissioning is at the heart of radical service change. Training and greater awareness about dual diagnosis is as crucial among commissioners as it is among frontline staff. Primary Care Trusts (PCTs) are playing an increasingly important role but must be equipped to commission effectively.

Commissioners and providers should be aware of the nature and scale of the problem so that services are planned and resources targeted appropriately. Guidance on dual diagnosis in mental health inpatient and day hospitals recommends that 'commissioning agencies need to ensure that the assessment and treatment of substance misuse is addressed in all mental health service agreements and contracts'[6] – and the same should be true for mental health services with regard to substance misuse. Contracts with providers should acknowledge the work done by a range of agencies, which may not be running explicitly dual diagnosis services. Typically, the extent or nature of an underlying mental health problem may only come to light when a person is receiving support for their substance misuse and vice versa. It may be appropriate for staff to continue to work with them, but the need for additional input from specialist services and increased staff time should be adequately resourced.

Whilst there is a need for more funding, the answer lies not only in more money but in using existing resources more intelligently. Although funding may come from different streams, it must be adequate, secure and long-term. We would like to see greater emphasis on funding following the person along their care pathway, according to their changing needs.

WORKFORCE, TRAINING AND PROFESSIONAL ROLES

Working with people who have dual diagnosis is inherently challenging, as it naturally requires a knowledge of both mental health and substance use. This is understandably daunting. The Dual Diagnosis Capability Framework is helpful in several respects.[7] It recognises that training is needed on different levels and that it is not necessary for everyone to become experts, but it does draw attention to the breadth of professionals from different agencies, who require training. Secondly, its aim is not to impose new requirements but to bring together a range of different occupational standards into one framework. Significantly, it reflects that a capability includes a commitment to working with new models of professional practice and taking responsibility for life-long learning. In other words, attitudes, values and knowledge play a crucial role.

There are valuable training courses available and it is important that staff are released to attend. Training should not become a means to an end.

Ongoing supervision, regular time for reflective practice and continuing professional development are equally important. This should start early, at pre-registration as well as post-registration of various occupations.

Working with people who have a dual diagnosis is challenging, but can also be rewarding, if staff have the right skills and feel confident about using them. There is also a balance to be struck between professionals continuing to work with individuals and not automatically deferring to the 'specialists', and knowing when it is most appropriate to refer. As one of Turning Point staff member in a community drug project has said, 'informing other professionals about what services are on offer, where they are based and how to refer, can be as valuable as drug and alcohol awareness'.

In our opinion, a workforce that is equipped to work with dual diagnosis should be built on three foundations. Professional competence, as outlined above, is one, but the other two are more challenging to bring about: appropriate work practices and a positive, can-do attitude.

Changing professional ways of working and looking beyond professional labels

Although practice is changing, a continued insistence that one problem – whether substance misuse or mental ill-health – be sorted out before the other is addressed, is unhelpful.

Whilst there is a place and role for diagnosis, this should be the vehicle for addressing a person's needs and not a barrier to receiving help. In the same way, while there is a need for clinical specialists and other professional roles, professional labels should enhance the skill mix required and not undermine it. Having the competence to serve the client group is more important than professional labels.

There should also be a healthy respect for different disciplines and also for the expertise which different sectors bring, i.e. both voluntary and statutory. The diverse nature of individuals and the challenges they present mean that no one sector has all the answers.

Changing attitudes and values

Sometimes, workers do have the appropriate skills but are reluctant to engage with 'difficult' or time-consuming clients. There are many reasons why a service user may perceive their issues differently from a practitioner. Some people may not acknowledge the presence or extent of their difficulties or they may not see their substance misuse or mental health as presenting so much of a problem as do other challenges in their lives. Different cultural, ethnic and religious perspectives should also be taken into account.

PROVISION FOR BLACK AND MINORITY ETHNIC COMMUNITIES

Currently service provision is poor for members of black and minority ethnic (BME) communities. We do not conclude this simply as a result of our own observations. Census studies by the Mental Health Act Commission have shown wide disparities in the comparative experience of service provision, level of choice and outcomes for those from BME communities. Similarly, the Sainsbury Centre report *Breaking the Circles of Fear*[8] and the inquiry into the death of David Bennett[9] are objective and indisputable testaments to continuing inequality of access in services for BME groups. This is firstly a legal breach of obligations in the Race Relations Amendment Act to ensure best practice and foster good race relations. But the obligation is not only legal. The issue points to a more profound problem in social care provision: that a poor quality service for BME communities is generally a poor quality service for everyone else.

The experience of these communities demonstrates the need for a shift in the delivery of mental health services. The Department of Health's *Delivering Race Equality in Mental Health Care*[10] is a five-year programme to improve outcomes for people from BME backgrounds, and the inclusion of dual diagnosis practice is an essential plank in it. Addressing a person's co-existing mental health, substance use and other needs requires effective coordination and inter-agency working, and so presents the impetus for change in service provision, both for BME groups and for everyone else as well.

Working explicitly with diverse, complex and often conflicting values between professionals and service users, underpins all practice. In dual diagnosis, where shared decision-making includes a range of vastly different perspectives and beliefs, and where there are no obvious and simple answers, working with values is essential. The value-based practice methods developed by Professor Bill Fulford at the University of Warwick and the seminal analysis in *The Oxford Textbook of Philosophy and Psychiatry*[11] examine in detail the methodology of using values assumptions explicitly as a helpful tool in diagnosis. The alternative to this kind of approach is that of allowing assumptions about values to be hidden deep within decision-making, and consequently only surfacing in the disproportionate nature of treatment for those within BME communities. Such work is essential to our understanding of social care and mental health and has particular relevance to dual diagnosis work.

SERVICE DELIVERY

Measurement of results or outcomes – what matters?

In this target-driven culture, it is impossible to escape targets and these have their place, but only if they result in improved service delivery on the front line. Service performance must measure what matters to the people with co-existing mental health, substance use and other needs who are using services. Conversations with committed professionals identify some of the perverse incentives built into the current systems. For example, funding is often justified by the number of people using a service rather than by the quality of that contact, or evaluations of service performance seldom record the small steps which are required to reach the bigger goal.

Improving coordination

The Care Programme Approach (CPA) is a key vehicle to improving multi-agency working. Whatever arrangements are made, there must be clarity about roles, responsibilities and referral routes. We strongly advocate CPA having statutory force, so that there is an obligation both to follow its principles and for local authorities and others to provide what has been outlined in the plan.

Person-centred services

Due to the breadth of need, people with a dual diagnosis present to a whole host of agencies including GPs, A&E, criminal justice settings, housing providers, voluntary agencies, mental health, substance use or social services.

There must be better links not only between primary and secondary services, but also between mainstream social care services. Within a professional's specialist expertise or distinct areas of activity, they should be aware of how their role fits into the matrix of others and how they complement the work of others.

There is a great need for services in the community such as those run by Turning Point. Support Link provides intensive community support to people with severe mental health problems and other issues including offending behaviour and substance misuse. Housing Link offers practical and emotional support for people who are at risk of losing their tenancy as a result of a mental health problem, learning disability or drug or alcohol difficulty.

CASE STUDY

When referred to Support Link, Diane had schizophrenia, misused amphetamines and had a history of non-engagement with services. Her daughter had been taken into care. Her project worker visited her whilst in hospital and, on discharge, Diane's priority was to re-establish contact with her daughter. Initial support focused on repaying debts and managing her tenancy and, over time, accessing the local drug project and other community services. Diane has been clean for many months and now has her daughter living with her at home again.

Treatment outcomes are improved if a person is engaged with treatment and that may involve achieving stability in other areas before more 'clinical' therapeutic work can commence. Working with dual diagnosis should be practical as well as clinical. For example, Mike, who has bipolar disorder, was threatened with eviction due to an overgrown garden and neglect of his home, so discussing a reduction of his alcohol intake took second place to sorting out the immediate problem.

It is also important to develop a more consistent understanding and common language around dual diagnosis.

We welcome the emphasis on choice and person-centred approaches in many areas of healthcare. It is essential that these concepts are not mere rhetoric, but also become reality for those who may be perceived as being more difficult. People with a dual diagnosis are challenging to current systems as they are illustrate a common problem experienced in many other areas of practice – that as the severity, nature and combination of an individual's needs vary, they each require a range of different services, at different levels.

Person-centred services are flexible and designed around what individual service users consider to be important from their *own* perspective. Services endeavour to adapt and change to reflect the needs of current clients. For Turning Point, having a person-centred approach is about the culture and values of the service. As a large social care charity, Turning Point does not underestimate the scale of the task, but it is a goal that we must all work towards.

EXAMPLE

The ethos underpinning Crisis Point, a 24/7 mental health crisis support centre run by Turning Point in Manchester, is to actively support people within their definition of crisis and its impact on their lives. Clients can choose whether to stay in the six-bed unit or to use the external non-residential service. Jane comments, 'I can access similar services, but it's much more convenient as I have a young son.'

Those with dual diagnoses have an inherent understanding of the complexity of their needs. The current standard of service is not meeting their needs, and they know it. In many cases, they have turned to self-medication as a solution to the problem. Engaging service users is the only way to achieve a long-term and sustainable outcome for those with dual diagnosis. This is a challenge in social engagement, in mental well-being and in mental health. Similarly, dual diagnosis is not just a challenge for professionals, but for service users as well. The solution is in acknowledging the expertise of the service user's contribution within the structure of their professional treatment.

At the beginning of this chapter, we said that it is too easy to diagnose clinically, by using a system of classification such as the *Diagnostic Statistical Manual* or the International Classification of Diseases. We all know that this is meaningless if it cannot translate diagnosis into a meaningful exchange with the patient. Dual diagnosis, in our opinion, presents an 'excuse remover' to those services and professionals who seek to reduce complexity to convenience. However, it could present us with a new vision for mental health within the paradigm of a social care system centred around a person's whole needs, rather than just the delivery of a single solution.

Dual diagnosis, although complex, is a good demonstration of the law that the complexity of an issue tends to fill the space left by its inherent simplicity. Essentially, it's about people who aren't very different from you or me.

The authors would like to thank service users and staff at Turning Point for their help, particularly Support Link and Crisis Point.

REFERENCES

1 Lehman A, *et al.* 1989. Cited by Weaver T. *Dual Diagnosis: the co-morbidity of psychotic mental illness and substance misuse.* London: The Centre for Research on Drugs and Health Behaviour; 1999 (No. 63).
2 Banerjee S, Clancy C, Crome I, editors. *Dual Diagnosis Information Manual – co-existing problems of mental disorder and substance misuse.* London: The Royal College of Psychiatrists; 2002.
3 Weaver T, Madden P, Charles V, *et al.* Co-morbidity of substance misuse and mental illness collaborative study. *Br J Psychiatry.* 2003; **183**: 304–13.
4 Department of Health. *Dual Diagnosis Good Practice Guide.* Mental Health Policy Implementation Guide. London: Department of Health; 2002.
5 Care Services Improvement Partnership. *Autumn Assessment: dual diagnosis in mental health.* Completion Notes. London: CSIP; 2006.
6 Department of Health. *Dual Diagnosis in Mental Health Inpatient and Day Hospital Settings.* London: Department of Health; 2006.
7 Hughes L. *Closing the Gap.* A capabilities framework for working effectively with people with combined mental health and substance use problems (dual diagnosis).

Centre for Clinical and Academic Workforce Innovation (CCAWI). University of Lincoln; 2006.

8 Sainsbury Centre for Mental Health. *Breaking the Circles of Fear.* London: The Sainsbury Centre for Mental Health; 2002.

9 Norfolk, Suffolk and Cambridgeshire Strategic Health Authority. *Independent Inquiry into the Death of David Bennett.* Cambridge: SHA; 2003. Available at: www.nscstha. nhs.uk/4856/11516/David%20Bennett%20Inquiry.pdf.

10 Department of Health. *Delivering Race Equality in Mental Health Care: an action plan for reform inside and outside services and the government's response to the independent inquiry into the death of David Bennett.* London: Department of Health; 2005. Available at: www.dh.gov.uk/assetRoot/04/10/07/75/0410075.pdf.

11 Fulford B, Thornton T, Graham G, editors. *Oxford Textbook of Philosophy and Psychiatry.* Oxford: Oxford University Press; 2006.

CHAPTER 7

Advocacy: does it really work?

ROBERTA WETHERELL and ANDREW WETHERELL

The authors have had a wide experience of developing advocacy services in different mental healthcare settings. While the concept of advocacy itself is not new, the recognition of the need to establish effective advocacy services to support and inform service users during treatment, and to help them express their reactions and share them with the staff who treat them, is comparatively recent. Advocacy is establishing itself as a significant feature in contemporary mental healthcare.

INTRODUCTION

Advocacy is not a new concept; in fact, it has been around in one form or another for a significant time. Within mental health services, it has, of course, been visible since at least the mid-1980s. Interestingly, as pointed out by the late Professor David Brandon,[1] advocacy actually dates back nearly 400 years – in 1620, a pamphlet titled *The Petition of the Poor Distracted People in the House of Bedlam* was published. It is probable that the pioneer of advocacy was John Perceval. At the age of nine, his father, a Tory prime minister, was assassinated and John became 'mentally ill', which resulted in his being shut away in private mental institutions for a number of years. In the mid-1840s, Perceval was responsible for founding the Alleged Lunatics Friends' Society and this organisation advocated for people in the asylums as well as campaigning the Government on relevant issues.[2]

Despite over 20 years of modern-day mental health advocacy projects, this essential service can still be seen struggling for recognition, understanding and appropriate resources all around the United Kingdom (UK). In particular, there can often be problems in achieving a 'shared understanding' between all relevant parties of what advocacy is, how it works, its boundaries and the significant advantages of having such a service available locally.

In addition, appropriate funding and commissioning arrangements, as well as achieving good working relationships between advocates and staff, can also prove to be problematic. It is therefore rewarding to find approaches where the above issues have been addressed. Where this happens and a pragmatic and professional approach is adopted, the resulting service is usually of immense benefit to all those concerned. The value of independent support and provision of balanced information is immeasurable but absolutely vital and must, therefore, be properly recognised, supported and commissioned for the benefit of service users and practitioners alike.

Whilst there is a lot of good work being delivered by advocacy projects around the UK, provision of this service is still quite patchy. This, we suggest, is due in the main to inadequate funding arrangements and unrealistic expectations which all too often set the service up to fail. The lack of robust and supportive commissioning arrangements can directly lead to unfocused, poorly coordinated and sometimes irresponsible advocacy service provision. Sadly, therefore, good practice tends to be all too uncommon, and independent advocacy service providers across the UK tend to experience similar problems.

SUPPORTING EFFECTIVE ADVOCACY

Poor quality support and supervision often lead to problems for both the service and the client. Service users will usually ask for help with highly emotive issues for both themselves and the advocate. This may lead to boundaries being blurred and advocates finding themselves making judgements about the client, the issue, or perhaps both. Because the issues being addressed can be emotionally demanding, the lack of good quality support and supervision often leads to burn-out for the advocate. We recommend that all advocates have access to regular independent support sessions, and these should be provided by an appropriate individual who is external to the organisation, on at least a monthly basis. The financial implications in this respect should, of course, be factored into any funding application – this is something to look out for if you are a service commissioner, as it can demonstrate that the applying organisation understands key elements needed to support a successful project.

Sometimes the provider agency itself might not be an appropriate provider of advocacy. The battle for funding in non-statutory agencies has led to some organisations seeing the management of advocacy projects as a way of raising much-needed revenue by recruiting advocates and then charging management fees. Whilst some organisations clearly have very good track records of project management in general, it does not mean that they have an understanding of the issues facing advocates. Support and supervision may then become inadequate and the project becomes at best ineffective, at worse a risk. Although these organisations often offer management at cheaper rates, we would argue that this is false economy as specialist knowledge is vitally important if the project is to be successful.

Quality support, supervision, ongoing training and the like need to be reflected in the budget, and it is important that service commissioners show they are committed to financing quality services by making sure these areas are embedded within Service Level Agreements which, of course, helps to ensure the best value from the investment.

Training is another area which needs to be monitored and properly funded by service commissioners. Advocates require training in areas such as confidentiality, boundary setting, the Mental Health Act and associated legislation, how services relate to each other, treatment options, basic understanding of benefits and housing issues. Whilst the list can be almost endless, the important thing for the advocates is to know when to seek specialist advice for dealing with complicated cases. Specialist training for advocates working in secure services with very risky clients is crucial, as these advocates will need to understand security procedures together with some of the clinical issues. They will also have to work more closely with the clinical team, particularly with high-risk patients. (The area of secure mental health advocacy is addressed later in the chapter.)

When there is a successful advocacy project, the benefits for all involved are well worth both the effort and cost. Until recently, psychiatry was a branch of medicine that gave patients little information and even less choice. The early pioneers of advocacy in mental health services challenged this by sharing information, telling patients what treatments might be an option and encouraging patients to question decisions made about them without consultation. At the same time, the service user movement became active by campaigning for the rights of people with mental health problems, including their right to exercise choices and take some control of their lives. Although they initially met with opposition from mental health workers, this is changing with staff now seeing the benefits of working towards informed compliance (or concordance) rather than forced treatment.

For many staff, this way of working is not only easier, but also quite rewarding as patients are much happier, have a better quality of life and move on to independent living with or without service support much more quickly.

Service users who are empowered, properly consulted, well informed and make their own choices also report a much-improved quality of life. Advocates have an holistic approach to the clients' issues, realising that housing, benefits, employment and social life are just as important as medication and treatment options. Helping people to address all of these issues improves their equality of opportunities in life.

Group advocacy (patients' councils or service user forums) is another area which advocacy providers are often asked to facilitate. We see no problem with this, providing roles for the workers are very clear. We believe that a separately funded position of 'service user involvement worker' is the only way to ensure that boundaries are not blurred between one-to-one advocacy and group advocacy–service user participation. The service user involvement worker should only be dealing with service-related issues which affect many service users or certain groups of service users – not individual issues. Points raised by service user forums can make an extremely useful contribution to service development by helping to ensure that services are both responsive to service users' needs and effective in meeting those needs. The service user involvement worker position should be funded in its own right, and by employing someone with this very specific remit, services can ensure that a representative service user voice can be heard in all aspects of service planning and development. Clearly, this helps prevent the old cry of 'pet service users' and 'maverick service users', and concerns of non-representative views being put forward.

SOME KEY POINTS FOR EFFECTIVE ADVOCACY PROVISION

➤ Realistic funding must be made in relation to the service required. We suggest that service commissioners should be looking to allocate an appropriate annual figure per potential client, taking into account the service setting and needs of the client group.
➤ Appropriate and accessible policies and procedures are essential, including realistic approaches to confidentiality, e.g. on first contact with a client, the advocate clearly explains that confidentiality will be breached if significant issues of risk arise which affect the service user and/or others.
➤ Adequate support and supervision (including external support) are vital for advocates.
➤ Regular support and clinical supervision must be made for advocacy project managers.
➤ Functional office accommodation is necessary, ideally within easy reach of service users.

➤ Proactive as well as reactive service delivery should be envisaged. Advocates need to make themselves available on the wards and have proactive approaches towards the more disempowered, excluded and vulnerable patients.

➤ Regular meetings need to be scheduled with commissioning staff and senior management from the service providers in order to discuss emerging themes and issues of concern so that these may be quickly addressed by the relevant parties.

➤ Effective engagement protocols need to be devised, covering issues in relation to the advocacy service interface with care providers.

➤ Robust and effective service level agreements need to be made with service commissioners.

➤ Appropriate record-keeping is required – covering, for example, the type and duration of contacts with service users as well as issue categories and the type of service user engaging the service.

➤ Active monitoring of the above data by service commissioners needs to occur, as well as performance management in relation to the service level agreement. The University of Durham Review[3] of advocacy service provision at Ashworth High Security Hospital provides good evidence-based recommended approaches to developing effective advocacy which are applicable to service provision whatever the setting. Therefore, this document can be a valuable resource to service commissioners. Achieving high quality and consistent service provision is, of course, the ultimate goal and this will be achieved by ensuring responsible and supportive commissioning approaches towards independent advocacy service provision.

➤ Regular advocacy training for service users and staff needs to be delivered by workers from the advocacy service in order to ensure a shared understanding of what independent advocacy is and how it works.

➤ As far as possible, advocacy services should be totally independent of care providers. The authors suggest that advocacy services should be independently financed.

➤ Good advocacy provision should take pressure from practitioners, who often carry out various advocacy-related tasks such as chasing up solicitors, obtaining information on housing and dealing with benefits problems.

➤ There should be a senior management member as a link person for advocacy personnel, so that important issues can be addressed in a swift and effective fashion.

➤ A healthy tension between the advocacy service, care providers and service commissioners often means that advocacy is doing a good job, as, of course, part of the advocate's role is to highlight failures and shortcomings.

➤ An external independent review of advocacy service provision needs to occur at appropriate point(s) during the contract period.

➤ An ultimate goal of self-advocacy for all clients of the advocacy service should be envisaged.

WHO MAKES A GOOD ADVOCATE AND WHAT QUALITIES DO THEY NEED?

An issue that has been debated at length and will probably continue to be is that of whether an advocate must be a past or present mental health service user. The authors feel that this topic has parallels with the saying: 'There is a little bit of good in the worst of us and a little bit of bad in the best of us', in that we believe there are indeed some excellent service user advocates, and also some quite poor ones. A significant number of service users feel that having an advocate who has experienced mental health problems can be most helpful – and empathy is, of course, priceless – but there are some superb non-service user advocates out there doing a great job, too.

Regardless of the individual's background, we believe the following are some of the essential qualities which make a good advocate:[4]

➤ the ability to be clear-thinking and firmly on the patient's side
➤ a non-judgemental attitude towards patients
➤ a knowledge of mental health legislation
➤ good listening and communication skills
➤ the ability to set and keep effective boundaries
➤ patience
➤ the ability to keep one's own agenda firmly to one side
➤ a good support network for off-loading and use as a sounding board.

SOME CONSIDERATIONS FOR SPECIALIST ADVOCACY AREAS

Forensic/secure

Although advocacy services in the three English High Security Hospitals (Ashworth, Broadmoor and Rampton) are well established, advocacy projects for medium- and low-security units are still very much in their infancy. There are no generally accepted standards for the provision of advocacy in these types of setting or for this particular client group. Contracts for these services must therefore be very specific and detailed, outlining exactly what is expected of the advocacy service, including working protocols and the boundaries and limitations of the advocacy service. If the contract is not specific, then this presents problems when trying to measure or monitor the quality of the service or to effectively manage either the service or the contract. Words like 'appropriate' should not be used in the context of service provision as these can be interpreted in a wide variety of ways, for example saying that there should be 'appropriate' supervision. The contract should clearly state what supervision should be provided, including the frequency of supervision and who should be providing it. Similarly, phrases like 'undertake quality audit on a regular basis' are not specific enough as 'regular' could be interpreted as monthly or (at an extreme) every ten years, therefore the contract should give specific time spans between audits.

These services are so different from acute and community settings that the pure advocacy model is not appropriate for either secure settings or for users of secure services. There are special requirements of security that have to be taken into consideration, and whilst there is no suggestion that an advocacy service or an advocate might breach security, it is important for all concerned that the advocacy service not only abides by the security procedures but also understands the necessity for them – some measures may appear to be punitive and unjust, but they exist for very good reasons. There is also a similar issue about the client group and the reasons that they are deemed to be in need of high- or medium-security services rather than those of lower security. The chapter authors feel that some training around the clinical issues for this client group and also around risk assessment and risk management is vital for advocates who are going to work in secure settings or where the client group predominately have a forensic history. This is to protect both the advocate and the patients, and in some cases the staff working on the units.

The very complicated and specialised needs of forensic patients means that advocacy has to be delivered in quite a different way to acute or community settings. However, the basic principles of advocacy continue to apply. Whilst there still must be confidentiality for the patient concerned, there cannot be blanket confidentiality. In forensic services there has to be much more information exchange between the advocate and the clinical staff, including checking many of the issues with the clinical team before action is taken, especially if contacting outside agencies or persons is involved. As stated above, contracts for advocacy provision within secure services have to be much more specific and detailed than contracts for acute or community settings. Some clear protocols around boundaries should be drawn up to protect all parties. If these are not in place, it creates a possible risk for all concerned, including the most important person in this equation, the patient.

Advocates in secure settings should not be contacting outside agencies or persons directly (including the patient's family) without going through the clinical team or social work department, as it might be extremely damaging to do so and may even put the patient or others at risk. The limitations on the role of the advocate need to be clearly defined, as in other less secure care settings it is normal practice for the advocate to contact outside agencies or persons directly. The advocate should also be aware of any clinical reasons for requests not being met so that these can be explained to the patient.

The authors believe that a lack of information or perhaps a lack of understanding of the clinical concerns may lead to an advocate making some poorly informed decisions. Most of the problems can be avoided if the advocate and the service provider are properly prepared and the advocate has specific training for working in this type of environment. There also need to be clearly defined channels for challenging clinical decisions which the patient does not agree with.

In the same way that advocates need to be properly trained in clinical and security issues, staff working in secure services need to be properly prepared for advocacy. Whilst some members of staff have a very good understanding in this respect, others do not, and some do not welcome advocacy input. Some also find that advocacy is challenging and uncomfortable. However, effective advocacy services sometimes do need to be challenging, and this can create discomfort at times. If advocacy services were not challenging and questioning, there would be no point having them. This does not mean that the advocacy service should be confrontational, and at the same time neither should the service provider be defensive or obstructive to the advocate. Instead, there should at times be a healthy tension between the two parties.

Change can only happen if both parties are willing to work in a collaborative way to improve the quality of service delivery for patients, ensure that patients' views and concerns are heard and patients' rights are upheld. To enable this relationship between staff and the advocacy service to be a positive one, staff should undergo advocacy awareness training, and this needs to be ongoing from their induction.

Staff who have reservations about advocacy in secure services may feel differently if there are clear boundaries to the advocacy role and protocols drawn up to ensure consistent working practices. There needs to be a constant flow of information between the advocate and the clinical staff to ensure that any risk is minimised for all concerned. In practical terms it would mean that the advocate not only informs staff that they are on the ward but also who they intend to speak to so that they can be briefed if there are any clinical issues that day which they need to be aware of.

Support and supervision for the advocate is very important, especially in smaller medium-secure units where the advocate may well be working in isolation. Therefore, anyone who takes on this supervisory role needs to have an understanding of the complexities surrounding this type of service and the issues which might arise, as they can be very disturbing and take their toll emotionally.

Learning disabilities

Whilst specific tailored approaches are required in relation to all specialist areas, the following are some additional issues which may need to be considered in respect of effective advocacy engagement with patients who have learning disabilities:

➤ more time is usually needed for meaningful engagement and to explain issues
➤ translation of information into an easily understood format may be required
➤ advocates need gradually to build up effective working relationships with service users
➤ specialist types of communication may be needed, e.g. use of symbols and pictures as well as behaviour, expressions, etc.
➤ advocates may sometimes need to build up a knowledge of the service user from staff, relatives and/or friends.

SUMMARY

Whilst we have only covered forensic/secure in detail (leaving aside the many other specialist areas) and barely touched on learning disabilities, the authors hope that these examples help to highlight the need for advocacy services (tailored to the needs of the specific client group) in order to offer relevant independent support and information provision to some of the most vulnerable, disempowered and excluded individuals within the mental healthcare system.

ACHIEVING A SHARED UNDERSTANDING OF ADVOCACY

Without a doubt, achieving a shared understanding of advocacy between all interested parties is crucial in relation to establishing and maintaining an effective independent advocacy service. Therefore, training workshops for practitioners, service users and managers are vital in this respect.

Good guidance in this connection is included in the University of Durham's recommendations of good practice for 'Independent Specialist Advocacy'.[5]

However, the following may be a useful point of reference.

What advocacy is

➤ a free and individual service for every patient
➤ provision of balanced and impartial information
➤ support of patients in ward rounds, care planning meetings, etc.
➤ help for patients to voice their needs
➤ speaking for a patient if they cannot speak for themself
➤ supportive of self-empowerment
➤ always driven by a patient-defined agenda.

What advocacy is not

➤ a substitute for the complaints system
➤ directive towards patients
➤ a befriending service
➤ the giving of advice
➤ a tool to disrupt delivery of good quality care
➤ a replacement for social workers, solicitors or other professionals
➤ compulsory for patients to use
➤ a mechanism to replace effective processes for service user participation.

The benefits of advocacy

➤ improved quality of life for patients
➤ empowerment of individuals
➤ development of effective and responsive mental health services
➤ improved equality of opportunity
➤ reduced pressure on practitioners
➤ improved service delivery.

Once a shared understanding has been achieved, appropriately resourced independent advocacy can be highly effective for service users as well as practitioners. Patients may benefit greatly from the input of an advocate who can provide balanced information as well as one-to-one support in a range of settings. Additional benefits may include the lifting of pressure from practitioners once appropriate advocacy provision is in place.

In this context, it must be acknowledged that practitioners do, of course, advocate for patients. Indeed, some nurses' training originally promoted this as part of their professional role. However, if a practitioner takes the role of being the patient's advocate in the widest sense, sooner or later they will find themselves in a conflict of interest and this is an unreasonable expectation to be placed on any staff member. By having properly trained, supported and managed advocates available for patients, staff can concentrate on relevant clinical issues instead of having potentially to 'put their neck on the line' in an advocacy role.

A BRIEF VISION FOR THE FUTURE

Our ideal vision for the future would simply be for everyone who uses mental health services to be able to access independent advocacy services should they so wish. However, we have concerns about the currently changing legislation in respect of the Mental Health Act and the new Capacity Act. This could, in our view, lead to a two-tier system where, in the main, only patients who are covered by the above are able to access advocacy input due to the fact that advocacy services are prioritised and funded to address the needs of sectioned patients or those who lack capacity. Whilst these groups of vulnerable individuals obviously need a service, it should not be at the expense of the remaining service user population who may also have complex needs and have an equal right to access advocacy support.

Independent mental health advocacy services should be an integral part of today's mental healthcare. They bring an invaluable service to both patients and practitioners and must be adequately supported if we are to see them flourish in the 21st century.

REFERENCES

1 Brandon D. *Innovation Without Change?* London: MacMillan; 1991.
2 Hunter R, Macalpine I. John Thomas Perceval (1803–1876): patient and reformer. *Med Hist.* 1962; 6(4): 391–5.
3 Barnes D, Tate A. *Advocacy from the Outside Inside: a review of the patients' advocacy service at Ashworth Hospital.* Durham: University of Durham; 2000.
4 Wetherell A. Good advocacy: the vital ingredients. *Ment Health Pract.* 2000; 3(6): 9–11.
5 Barnes D, Brandon T, Webb T. *Independent Specialist Advocacy in England and Wales: recommendations for good practice.* Durham: University of Durham; 2002.

CHAPTER 8

Prejudice and progress

RORY HEGARTY and NUALA O'BRIEN

The authors, widely experienced in the field of communications and public relations, describe their work in a West London Mental Health Trust where they are attempting to counter and overturn the fears and negative images which swirl around mental illness – regularly described in our society with the use of prejudicial and pejorative language.

> 'When I start to get ill, all I have to do is walk down the street and it makes me worse. I see newspaper headlines about nutters and loonies. I see the way people look at me. By the time I get home, I'm in a dreadful state. I often end up in hospital again.'
>
> **Mental health service user, Hammersmith.**

People with mental ill-health face a prejudice that probably no other group in society has to contend with. While much has been done to tackle racism, sexism, homophobia and ageism, mental illness is routinely stigmatised in all walks of life – in the media, the community, by employers and even by some health and social care professionals. People are reluctant to admit to using mental health services either now or in their past, because they know that it is likely to create problems in their lives. This difficulty of getting service users to speak about their illness in a sense exacerbates the problem: it is difficult to challenge prejudice when its victims are justifiably unwilling to admit to experiencing mental ill-health.

Many service users say that the stigma of mental illness is almost as bad as the illness itself, the two feeding one another in a vicious cycle that makes recovery from illness extremely difficult. Eradicating such prejudice is increasingly a challenge being taken on by mental health charities, Trusts and service users themselves. It is an issue which has the power to galvanise all of these groups, and service users in particular – and there may lie the key to addressing it successfully.

AN ANNUAL GENERAL MEETING WITH A DIFFERENCE

> 60% of people said the risk of discrimination would prevent them telling someone about their own or another's mental distress.
>
> *Attitudes to Mental Health.* Department of Health; 2000.

Annual general meetings (AGMs) in the Health Service are notoriously dull events, where worthy and important information is communicated to a small group of staff and even fewer members of the public.

Recently, however, the West London Trust with which we are associated decided to take a different approach and try to liven up the AGM by turning it into the launch of a local campaign against stigma. This would support SHiFT, the national initiative launched by the Department of Health with the same purpose, developing a local campaign in which service users, carers, Trust staff, local schools, the media, employers and others could ultimately engage. The hope was that the issue might raise greater interest among service users in particular and boost the normally tiny AGM attendance.

What followed took us completely by surprise. People queued down the street to get into the venue, extra seating had to be hastily arranged and suddenly the meeting was packed to capacity. Users of our services had turned out in droves and, once there, they were going to have their say. One service user read out her poem about the prejudice she faced, others asked searching questions about the use of medication versus talking therapies.

MIRROR IMAGE by Anna Gabell

I have become a member of the Mental Tribe –
The warriors 'caste' out;
By fake shamen,
Who have enacted ritual humiliation on us.

Why were we told to leave the camp fires?
To pack up our wigwams –
And our old kit bags?
Was it because we were in possession of too much
And they were troubled by it?

We passed their initiation ceremonies
In our own abstract absence –
Isolated –
Beyond belief!

We must not blame our knowledge
On the greedy impoverishment
Of their naked eyes;
One of them looked at me the other day,
Inflicted a painful glance.
Does this mean that I have lost my powers of invisibility?

The Mental Tribe survives,
On tranced feet,
Our skins tattooed in sanity.
We have been disinherited
And have become spirited nightmares –
That Society's mirror will NOT allow –
On reflection.

> *Anna Gabell read one of her poems at the launch of West London SHiFT*
> *Reproduced with permission.*

The usual moribund AGM was a million miles away as the meeting sparked lively debate, passionate interjections and often tumultuous applause. Here, clearly, was an issue with which service users could identify and an issue they wanted the Trust to do something about. In the weeks that followed, service users and staff contacted us on a daily basis, asking about the anti-stigma campaign and how they could get involved. It was not just an encouraging launch for our campaign, it was something of a revelation.

MAKING A START

> 'I have been upset by the reaction of people with me when I'm mentally ill. It's another extra burden on top of a very traumatic and hideous illness.'
>
> **Sylvie**

The stigmatisation of mental ill-health is a daunting issue. Myths and prejudice are everywhere and beginning to tackle them can look like an impossible task. When we decided to launch a local campaign, we knew we were one small voice in one pocket of the country trying to take on a prejudice which is deep-seated and frequently reinforced by lurid media headlines about the rare cases where people with mental illness have committed violent crimes.

There are a number of similar projects elsewhere in the United Kingdom and most of these are feeding into the national SHiFT campaign or the work being done by mental health charities. On their own, these projects will hopefully make a small difference, but they will not change the world.

Our aim, therefore, was to make a start – to make our own small contribution to challenging stigma. Our West London SHiFT campaign aims to work alongside existing projects in the Trust around social inclusion, particularly employment, as well as other national initiatives. It has four initial elements:

➤ our *Write Now* campaign – based on *See Me*, a similar campaign run in Scotland with great success – encouraging service users, carers, staff and supporters to challenge stigma in the media
➤ a schools project involving local school children and teachers in projects around mental ill-health and stigma
➤ promotion of positive images and stories around mental ill-health
➤ close links to the national campaign and close work with Mental Health Trusts and charities in support of the anti-stigma agenda.

These are modest objectives, each requiring a good deal of work.

THE WRITE NOW CAMPAIGN

'You never read "crazy person gets job and becomes well, marries and has children".'

Patricia

The aim of this campaign is simple – to create a group of local people prepared to actively challenge the stigmatisation and misreporting of mental health in the national and local media. It also has the potential to expand to a wider online campaigning network.

The campaign will work along the lines pioneered by Amnesty International and other charities, who have encouraged their supporters to write and challenge perceived injustices. If a newspaper editor receives a letter from the Trust complaining about an article, it may not have a huge impact – but imagine the impact if the editor received 20 or 30 letters.

Any stigmatisation of mental illness is to be challenged. Such stigmatisation might include use of derogative terms like 'psycho' and 'loony' in relation to mental illness; articles implying that most mentally ill people are a danger to others; use of mental illness as a label, e.g. 'Schizophrenic Fred Bloggs attacked and killed a neighbour'; and any suggestion that people who have mental ill-health are somehow less able to do a job or play a part in their community. We have set up a team of media monitors – Trust staff and volunteers – who will look out for offending articles and alert the group by email or phone. Model letters of complaint will be developed as part of a toolkit for supporters.

MEDIA 'MADNESS'

60% of people with mental health problems blame media coverage for the discrimination that they face in their daily lives. 40% of the general public associate mental illness with violence and say that this belief is based on the media. 64% of journalists say that media coverage of mental health could be improved.

> **West London Mental Health NHS Trust.** *Challenging Stigma,*
> *Changing Lives.* **West London Mental Health NHS Trust; 2006.**
> **Citing Mental Health Media; 2001.**

SCHOOLS PROGRAMME

'Friends dropped me because I had a mental illness. They had young children and maybe they thought I would harm them. And that really upset me.'

Lydia

There have been a number of attempts to engage school children in mental health issues, including a notable national project by the Samaritans which provides lesson plans for teachers to discuss these issues. The stigma theme also sits nicely alongside the anti-bullying agenda now common to all state schools.

One of the biggest challenges we face as a Trust is the scope of any project to engage local schools – we cover three London boroughs (Ealing, Hammersmith–Fulham and Hounslow), as well as Broadmoor Hospital in Berkshire. Our schools programme is therefore being launched initially in one borough – Ealing – with the aim of gradually expanding to take in the rest of our localities.

The ultimate aim is to develop a vibrant project which involves service users, consultant psychiatrists, nurses and other staff visiting schools to talk about mental health as an issue – and as a potential area of employment for young people. We envisage this programme growing until it includes all of the following:

➤ a mental health awareness pack for schools
➤ competitions for local school children with a mental health theme – for instance in public speaking, creative writing or designing a poster
➤ partnerships with the voluntary sector and/or the local press around these competitions
➤ recruitment information being sent to schools/colleges
➤ work experience placements
➤ related drama and art projects
➤ links with private sector sponsors.

This ambitious undertaking got off to a good, if modest, start when students from Elthorne Park High School in Ealing performed a moving drama about bullying at the launch of our SHiFT campaign. We hope that this small step is the first on a long road towards real engagement and involvement of our local schools.

YOU'RE MORE LIKELY TO BE HIT BY A DRUNK THAN A MENTALLY ILL PERSON

Levels of violence among people abusing alcohol or drugs are far higher than levels of violence involving people with a severe mental illness. Of 873 homicides in 2002, fewer than 5% were attributable to mental illness. The frequency of such homicides has remained the same for 30 years, whilst the rate of homicides among the general population has significantly increased.

West London Mental Health NHS Trust. *Challenging Stigma, Changing Lives.* **West London Mental Health NHS Trust; 2006. Citing** *The National Confidential Inquiry into Suicide and Homicide by People With Mental Illness.*

'Everyone knows what it's like to so-called "lose it" – imagine what it's like if you were in that state for years.'

Patricia

PROMOTING THE POSITIVE

A key goal of mental health services is increasingly to challenge perceptions of mental illness by putting across more realistic images and telling people's stories. While many service users are understandably reluctant to tell their stories, it remains the case that the best myth-busting is done by the people who are victims of the myths. The Trust is therefore increasingly involving service users in its publications and other publicity and using statistics which challenge the myths.

An example is the supposed link between mental illness and violence. Only a very small number of mentally ill people are likely to be violent and the vast majority are more likely to be victims of attacks. Attacks by people who have been abusing alcohol and drugs are far higher in number. The Trust is developing a poster campaign around this theme, which it hopes to use locally in schools, workplaces and other community settings.

Another example is the idea that mental illness can't be cured. Mental ill-health is widely portrayed as permanent or at best recurring, yet mental disorders are treatable and as likely to respond favourably to treatment as are physical illnesses.

These themes were also taken up in our 2006 annual report, *Challenging Stigma, Changing Lives*, and will continue to be central to all of our public communications.

IT COULD BE YOU

One in six people will currently be experiencing problems with their mental health. That means that even if you haven't experienced a mental health problem yourself, you almost certainly know someone who has.

Mental illness is in many ways the last taboo. The myths, fears and prejudice surrounding it mean people often feel they need to keep it a secret because of the way others treat them. The media all too often reinforces prejudice by using negative and inaccurate stereotypes – in spite of the fact that some of our greatest politicians, academics, business brains and artists have proved that mental ill health need not be a barrier to success.

West London Mental Health NHS Trust. *Challenging Stigma, Changing Lives,* West London Mental Health NHS Trust; 2006. Citing Office for National Statistics. *Survey of Psychiatric Morbidity Among Adults Living in Private Households.* London: HMSO; 2000.

WORKING WITH THE NATIONAL CAMPAIGN AND OTHERS

'Being left behind by people has been extremely soul-destroying and has left me with worse illness over the years.'

Mark

It is important that we share learning and experience from our own and others' work as the five-year SHiFT programme progresses. With this in mind, we are closely monitoring the national programme and trying to reproduce some of the national work at a local level.

Clearly, the more individuals and organisations who get involved in anti-stigma initiatives nationwide, the more successful our campaign and other similar initiatives will be. It is, in a sense, a drop in the ocean – but one we hope is going in the same direction as the tide.

MIND YOUR LANGUAGE

Words like 'schizo' and 'psycho' are too often used by the media and elsewhere to inaccurately describe mental illness. Using guidelines drawn up by the national SHiFT campaign, we will be working with our local media to help them avoid such pejorative terms and to report mental ill health in a balanced way.

West London Mental Health NHS Trust. *Challenging Stigma, Changing Lives.* West London Mental Health NHS Trust; 2006.

WORKING WITH EMPLOYERS

'I had a job with a small company in London. I had to go in to hospital and when my boss found out it was a mental hospital, I was told the job was no longer available.'

Patricia

One of the themes that emerged at our successful campaign launch was that many users of mental health services feel that whatever contribution they may make as advocates for themselves or others as part of Trust and other projects, paid work for any people with mental ill-health remains extremely difficult to get.

Indeed, statistics show that people with mental illness are more likely to be unemployed than people with any other disability. This is due to prejudice rather than their own capacity – obviously, people who are severely mentally incapacitated and unable to work would not be expected to do so. Fewer than 40% of employers say they would employ someone with a mental illness, while 75% of employers say that employing someone with schizophrenia would be impossible or very difficult.[1]

Alongside our SHiFT initiative, West London Mental Health Trust has established a major project to work with local employers around mental health. Not only are we revising our own employment procedures to ensure they reflect best practice, but we are approaching others to ask them to do the same. An emerging theme for our next AGM is that of employment – getting employers to sign up to a charter saying that they are open to employing people with mental ill-health – and getting service users and carers to share their good and bad experiences of paid work.

One initiative that had a great impact involved Queens Park Rangers Football Club, who organised training sessions for service users. The link between physical and mental health is well known and a number of service users felt that their condition was improved as a result of the training experience and other related physical activity.

GETTING A JOB IS A JOB IN ITSELF

People with mental health problems have the highest rate of unemployment among people with disabilities. One important part of the social inclusion agenda is the employment of people with mental health problems and other disability, both within and outside of the Trust. Another is to ensure that our current service users have a clear pathway, as part of their recovery, to employment and vocational opportunities. An employment charter will be produced to clearly state what we aim to do to support this agenda, together with our partnership organisations.

West London Mental Health NHS Trust. *Challenging Stigma, Changing Lives.* **West London Mental Health NHS Trust; 2006. Citing 'Hitting the wall',**
The Guardian; **5 July 2006.**

HURDLES TO OVERCOME

'The lunatics are making over the asylum' – newspaper headline about the proposed redevelopment of Broadmoor Hospital.

Daily Mirror, **13 March 2006.**

As our campaign develops, we are aware that there are a number of obstacles to its success and that of the wider anti-stigma movement.

Figures recently released by the Government suggested that one murder a week was committed by someone with a mental illness. The result was a series of newspaper headlines about the dangers we face and why the Government's proposed Mental Health Act was desperately needed. But the figures require context. There are on average 52 murders a year by people who are mentally ill. This accounts for only 5% of all homicides[2] and that figure has remained static for the past 30 years.[3] While the debate about containing people who are a risk to others will go on, it is misleading to suggest that there is an increased risk of many people's worst fear – being murdered at random by a stranger who is mentally ill. (Indeed, the vast majority of murders are committed by someone known to the victim.)

Such bursts of publicity are a big challenge to the growing movement to tackle stigma. They reinforce prejudice that is already ingrained. This presents a challenge also for the Government. While on the one hand the Department of Health is sponsoring a campaign to eradicate prejudice, on the other it is putting out statistics which are likely to see that prejudice increase. What all of this indicates, however, is that mental health is on the agenda like never before, which represents a real opportunity to change perceptions.

Another big challenge we face in tackling stigma remains getting service users involved in the campaign. As part of our SHiFT campaign, we produced a short video in which service users talked about their experiences of stigma. Finding service users to take part was not easy. Many were willing to discuss what the content of the film should be and even to suggest others to take part, but they did not want to feature in it themselves. One person who did agree to participate was happy to talk about mental health in general, but reluctant to share his own experiences. It is to be hoped that as the anti-stigma movement gathers pace, more people will feel able to share their experiences without fearing the impact it may have on their lives.

A big obstacle in working with young people in schools is the prevalence of bullying and social exclusion as a result of peer pressure. Many young people want to exclude others and be part of a clique – teasing and isolating others can almost be a part of their identity. Indeed, this was one of the key lessons of the Liverpool Help Project, which ran a programme in local secondary schools. It is therefore important that those working with schools ensure that they are developing relationships and ongoing contact, rather than simply providing one-off lectures or lesson plans. Support also needs to be available through Child and Adolescent Mental Health Services (CAMHS), as some children will want to discuss their own experiences and mental health issues.

The biggest obstacle of all remains the widespread misunderstanding of mental illness. While this is often fuelled by abject media coverage, it would be a mistake to think that media coverage is exclusively responsible. While terms like 'nutter', 'psycho' and 'schizo' may have originated in the tabloids, it is fair to say that they are in widespread use and not always in the context of mental illness. Stuart Pearce, a former England footballer and ex-manager of Manchester City, took some pride in his on-field nickname of Psycho. People regularly describe friends as 'mad' or 'a nutcase' as a kind of compliment – it means they are funny and entertaining company. It is not within the scope of our campaign or any other to attempt to address the language of everyday life; rather, we need to ensure that offensive terms are not used in the context of mental illness.

A specific challenge faced by West London Mental Health Trust is that of challenging the stigma faced by that most vilified group of service users: patients in Broadmoor Hospital. In common with Ashworth and Rampton, Broadmoor is regularly described as a prison and its patients (or 'inmates') as monsters. While many Broadmoor patients have committed terrible crimes, they have usually done so whilst suffering severe mental illness. It is not acceptable to label them in such offensive language. Only a wider understanding of mental illness – and a bigger challenge to the tabloid notion of 'evil' – can begin to change this view. This is likely to remain an uphill struggle.

The Press Complaints Commission has issued guidance to journalists covering mental illness. This helpful guidance – including an emphasis that high-security hospitals are not prisons and that terms like 'schizo' and 'nutter' are not acceptable – is a welcome step forward. It is possible that, in spite of the obstacles outlined above, challenging the stigma of mental illness is an issue whose time has come.

MENTAL ILLNESS CAN BE CURED

Many people believe mental disorders are incurable. They may even view some treatments, like antidepressants or psychotherapy, as useless or harmful – even though in many cases they have been proved to be effective. In fact, mental disorders are treatable and are as likely to respond favourably to medical and other treatments as many physical illnesses. But the stigma of mental illness can make it harder for sufferers to seek help and more difficult for other people to help them.

West London Mental Health NHS Trust. *Challenging Stigma, Changing Lives.* West London Mental Health NHS Trust; 2006. Citing Royal College of Psychiatrists' Changing Minds campaign.

THE NEXT STEPS

'Once you are diagnosed with a mental illness, there is a stigma against you for life.'

Lydia

This chapter outlines the actions being taken by one NHS Trust in one area of the country. There are several equally worthy initiatives nationally and locally, but we need many more. The challenges set out above are not easy to overcome and the growing anti-stigma movement will need to be innovative, resourceful and determined if it is to succeed.

The national SHiFT campaign is looking to encourage and support local projects such as ours and to work with mental health charities and others who support its aims. To succeed, the anti-stigma movement will also need to draw on the support of opinion formers – members of parliament, the police, journalists, employers' organisations, trade unions, health and social care professionals – and many others in the wider community. As our own campaign starts out, we know that it cannot succeed alone and that all of these influences will be crucial.

But all great movements to change public perception have to start somewhere. In the 1980s, campaigns which highlighted racism, sexism and homophobia were dismissed as 'political correctness'. While something of that attitude remains in the tabloids and elsewhere, bigotry against these groups is now regarded as beyond the pale.

The success or failure of our campaign and the wider anti-stigma movement will depend enormously on our ability to involve service users themselves in challenging prejudice. In West London, we have made a very positive start. The phone is still ringing and people are still asking how they can get involved. Ultimately, there has to be a tipping point where user involvement in such campaigns becomes easier because the stigma of mental illness is being effectively challenged. But that day is a long way off. Until mental ill-health is regarded in the same way as a broken leg, a dose of flu or, in more serious cases, cancer, the goals of the anti-stigma movement will not have been achieved. But the tide, we hope, is beginning to turn.

KEEPING IT ALL IN

Some of the service users and carers who featured in our annual report did not want to use their real names. Their fear of being stigmatised was too great.

In one survey, 60% of people said the risk of discrimination and stigma would prevent them telling someone about their own or another's mental distress. We look forward to a day when having a mental health problem is not something people feel they have to keep secret.

West London Mental Health NHS Trust. *Challenging Stigma, Changing Lives.* West London Mental Health NHS Trust; 2006. Citing *Attitudes to Mental Health*, Department of Health, 2000.

REFERENCES

1 Manning C, White PD. Attitudes of employers to the mentally ill. *Psychiatr Bull.* 1995; 19: 541–3.
2 National Confidential Inquiry. *Avoidable Deaths: five year report of the National Confidential Inquiry into suicide and homicide by people with mental illness.* London: The Stationery Office; 2006.
3 National SHiFT campaign.

CHAPTER 9

Clients as colleagues: part of the path to recovery?

DEBBIE SINGH

The gradual refocusing of the mental illness service from a professionally dominated sphere into a culture of shared care with user and carer is at the centre of this piece. Progress can still be quite tentative.

> 'I drank every day, from age 18 until 38, just to get me through. The alcohol helped control my anxiety and let me sleep. But my mood swings caused problems at home and at work, and I was eventually diagnosed with bipolar disorder. At first, I did nothing to help myself recover or control my illness. I continued to drink, got divorced, my kids wouldn't speak to me, and I went through so many jobs. But then I found three ingredients that put me on the road to recovery. I started visiting a psychiatrist regularly and took the medication she prescribed; I found another person with my illness that I could connect with; and I took control of my finances and my life rather than passing the buck to other people. I can't emphasise enough the importance of having another person who has suffered from a mental illness to help me through. He couldn't replace my psychiatrist and he didn't try. But he did signpost, support, and keep putting me on the right track. After all, he had 40 years as an "expert" with first-hand knowledge of my condition.'
>
> **52-year-old John from London**

John's heartfelt words describe how support from another service user helped him to live with bipolar disorder. Numerous other personal stories and research studies reinforce this view. Support from peers can make a significant difference to self-esteem,[1,2] symptoms,[3–6] satisfaction,[7] and use of health and social services[8–12] among people living with a myriad of mental health issues and their families.[13] Providing peer support can have benefits for service users, too.[14]

Support from peers can include advocacy, companionship, counselling, self-management education, and helping at drop-in centres and voluntary groups. But what happens when service users take on the role of case managers – when service users become paid or unpaid professional colleagues?

While involving users in mental health services is generally seen as worthwhile,[15] and government policy in England supports and encourages this,[16,17] the effects of involving users have not been thoroughly evaluated. This chapter summarises the evidence about former or current clients working as case managers for others and explores whether this innovation might be acceptable and feasible in England, based on feedback from professionals and service users.

PEER-LED CASE MANAGEMENT

'Case management' or 'care management' has been defined in many different ways. Definitions vary widely depending on the programme type, location and condition of focus. Broadly speaking though, the principle behind case management is for one person or one team to take responsibility for ensuring that a service user has access to 'the right care, in the right place, at the right time'. Case management involves facilitating access to appropriate medical, rehabilitation, social and support programmes; liaising with various services; advocacy; and monitoring that services meet people's needs. In England, various competencies and professional frameworks have been developed focusing on case management,[18] but rather than relating solely to professionals of a certain type, the term also lends itself to encompass any person or team that takes responsibility for supporting people to access services throughout a care pathway. This broader definition is used in this chapter.

From the 1960s, in England and in many other parts of the world, large psychiatric institutions began to close – with service users receiving support in community facilities or via outpatient services instead. In the 1970s, case management was developed as a way to help coordinate the wide range of services available for people with severe mental health issues in the community. Over the past three decades, case management has gained popularity as an approach for supporting people with complex mental and physical needs. However, in many fields of mental health, the outcomes of case management have been conflicting or less than positive.[19] In fact, a Cochrane review based on randomised controlled trials concluded that for people aged 18 to 65 years with severe mental disorders, case management had no significant advantages over standard care.[20]

On the other hand, there is emerging evidence that some forms of case management may have benefits and could be worth exploring further. One of these adaptations involves service users acting as case managers or case manager assistants for others with mental health issues.[21,22] This model has been trialled since the early 1990s, predominantly in the United States (US). Most such studies train current or former users of mental health services with serious psychiatric illness, including schizophrenia and bipolar disorder, or with addiction issues.

So what is the evidence about peer-led case management? Well, the short answer is that it is sparse and conflicting.[23,24] But accounts from clients who have been helped with this approach and studies published over the past 10–15 years suggest that this may be an avenue worth exploring further. We searched 17 electronic databases, contacted experts in the field, and hand-searched journals and conference proceedings for reviews, trials and observational studies available as at December 2006.

Summarising the evidence about peer-led case management is difficult, not least because there are so many different terms and definitions used. One study suggested that there are more than 30 different titles used throughout the world to describe a service user who serves as a bridge between peers and professional services.[25] Another difficulty is that most of the evaluations available are descriptive and do not include comparison groups. Furthermore, much of the evidence is from North America, which has very different healthcare systems and services compared with England.

That said, there are some positives. For instance, one randomised controlled trial in the US found that peer case managers were as effective as professional case managers in maintaining the stability of people with severe mental illnesses over a two-year period.[26] Numerous other studies have found no differences in outcomes between peer case managers and professional case managers, with the authors concluding that this may mean that clients can effectively provide mental health services as members of a case management team.[27-32]

Another US trial found that, compared with standard case managers, peer case managers were associated with better take-up of services among people with severe mental illness. In the first six months, service users thought that their peer case managers understood and accepted them better than did regular providers. The authors concluded that peer case managers may be able to engage with service users more quickly and encourage them to use the facilities available to them.[33] This 'engagement' hypothesis is supported by studies which found that service users were more likely to 'open up' to peer interviewers when evaluating services.[34,35]

Another quasi-experimental study with a control group examined whether employing mental health clients as case manager assistants improved outcomes for people with serious mental illness in the US. Compared with people who received case management from a professional alone, or case management from a professional with a non-client assistant, those with a peer case manager assistant reported more frequent contact with their case managers, better quality of life, fewer major life problems, and improved self-image and social support after six months.[36]

Other trials and observational studies suggest that peer-led services are accepted by service users and their families[37,38] and that professionals feel that peers can effectively coordinate resources.[39,40] The most consistent findings appear to be that peer-led case management or advisory services help others to access services and remain in contact with case management teams[41] and that peer-led services may be seen as being more welcoming or accepting than standard services.[42]

There have also been investigations of the benefits and challenges of becoming a case manager or service provider among clients themselves.[43-7] For instance, one descriptive study suggested that clients acting in professional roles experienced substantial benefits, including employment and personal development. But there were also numerous challenges, including the attitudes of clients and professionals; organisational structure, supervision, and training needs; and impacts on their own recovery.[48] On the other hand, another trial found that peer case managers were no more likely to show signs of stress, diminished self-esteem, or burnout compared with professional case managers.[49] A survey in Canada found that peers working as service providers tended to have equal or better job satisfaction compared with other employees[50] and further descriptive study in the US found that peers working as case manager assistants had good job retention rates and low personal hospital admissions.[51]

PART OF THE PATH TO RECOVERY?

There does seem to be some evidence to suggest that peer case management might be worth testing further. But would this work in the United Kingdom (UK)? To gain feedback about this we surveyed 100 professionals providing mental health services in the voluntary or health sectors or via local authorities. We contacted every local authority and strategic health authority in England, asking them to nominate a service provider to interview or take part in an anonymous postal questionnaire. Every organisation responded, and the response rate from nominated individuals was 96%.

We also conducted three discussion groups with service users in London, Birmingham and Cornwall. Twenty-three service users who visited a drop-in group or workshop hosted by the voluntary or statutory sector were invited to take part in discussion groups when they attended their regular session. Service users were living with psychiatric illnesses and addiction problems. There was a 100% participation rate. No incentives were offered.

The views of service users and staff reported here are by no means representative of service users and professionals throughout England, but the aim was to gain some indication of the acceptance of the concept of peer case managers among a targeted group and to explore whether those we spoke to felt this was an area worth trialling further.

The views of professionals and service users were remarkably similar in terms of the perceived benefits of peer case management. The most commonly perceived benefits among both service users and staff were:

➤ engagement with clients and ability to 'speak on their terms'
➤ greater understanding of the issues faced by clients
➤ role modelling and demonstration of the potential for positive outcomes
➤ and personal benefits for those training as peer case managers.

'A really good aspect of this type of intervention would be working with someone "just like me". There would be less stigma and people might feel more comfortable and engaged with the service if they felt they were getting help from a peer rather than a professional. We do our best, but there is inevitably some degree of judgement and stigmatisation in professional service provision.'

Community mental health team member from London

Repeatedly, service users said that they could see the benefits of having another person with a similar condition working alongside them on their path to recovery.

'Something like this would really have helped me. Having someone who is just like you to point you in the right direction and to explain things would be good. The professionals try hard but at the end of the day you can feel more confident if someone who has been through it all is guiding you. And I guess it also gives you hope because you can see that someone else has made it through, so you can too.'

31-year-old Alice from Cornwall

Both service users and staff thought there would be benefits for those trained as peer case managers.

> 'Imagine recovering from depression or addiction and then being trained to help others. It would be fabulous. Not only would you get all that training and end up with a job at the end of it, but think of the job satisfaction.'
>
> **Local authority home worker from Sussex**

However, while the substantive benefits listed were similar between staff and service users, service users were much more likely to feel strongly that peer case management was an option worth exploring further. Professionals, particularly those from the health service, appeared more concerned by the potential challenges with this approach.

The main perceived barriers among both service users and staff were:

➤ whether the service would be of a high enough standard to avoid serious risk

➤ whether there would be any risks for peer case managers themselves

➤ whether it would take too much time and funding to train service users fully

➤ whether there was adequate motivation to implement such schemes in England.

> 'I think this idea has potential, particularly for people with depression or less severe conditions. My main concern is whether the service would work in practice. Could clients cope with providing such an intensive service to someone else? What type of training and support would be on offer? The danger is that the case managers would need to be very closely supervised – which takes time and resources – or that they would not be monitored well enough and that could result in real risks.'
>
> **Psychologist from East Anglia**

Professionals in both managerial and frontline posts wanted to how peer case managers would fit in with community matrons and specialist mental health teams, and whether these would be competing services. Service users mentioned that professionals may feel threatened or may not respect the role of peer case managers.

> 'You know, my brother lives in Canada and he told me about something similar over there that really works. But I don't know about here. Maybe the professionals would guard their turf. Maybe they would see us as a threat.

Maybe they would think we could not do the job properly or that we would muck it up. But at the end of the day, it could be really good for the ones that provide the service and the ones receiving it. How will we know unless we try?'

67-year-old Elsie from Birmingham

Some professionals were extremely sceptical about the potential for service users to offer high-quality intensive services. Others worried about whether service users would receive enough training to do an 'intensive job' or whether such peer case managers could work only with people with a relatively low level of severity.

There were also many questions raised about whether acting as care managers would hinder a service user's own progress – or be a help. These are questions that the existing evidence cannot answer unequivocally.

'How would this fit in with the individual's own recovery? Case manager professionals train for years to help them gain the skills they need, yet working with clients still affects them. Just how would that work for a client themselves who's now being asked to take on the role of case managing someone else?'

Mental health service manager from Cumbria

Despite these concerns, nine out of 10 service users and seven out of 10 professionals strongly agreed that the concept of peer case managers could be considered further in England.

Once again, it is important to emphasise that these views are by no means generalisable, but they do suggest that among those we spoke to there was support to consider some of the issues involved in more detail. The professionals who did not think the concept was worth persuing were most likely to be frontline health services staff, whose main stated concern was that service users may not have the competencies required to provide a full case management service. The service users who were wary of peer case management were more likely to be worried about potential negative impacts on the peer case managers themselves.

'I wouldn't support it because there would not be enough training and it could screw you up to listen to someone else's problems if you weren't better yet. They might say there would be good training and help and that, but really there probably would not be so it's better to be safe than sorry.'

22-year-old Bobbie from London

WHERE TO FROM HERE?

Engaging clients as part of the professional team, or using other forms of peer support, is based on the belief that people who have faced adversity can offer encouragement and hope to others facing similar situations. This belief is increasingly accepted for people with a variety of issues, such as addiction, trauma, and long-term conditions, but the stigma and stereotypes attached to mental illness may have impeded attempts to develop such peer support systems within mental health services.[52]

Based on a review of readily available evidence and feedback from 123 service users and professionals in England, there seems to be some indication that this model could be worth exploring further. However, there is a need for more information about or consideration of:

➤ what type of people this approach might be most effective for
➤ exactly what peer case managers would be required to do (given so many varying definitions)
➤ who might be the best people to train as peer care managers, based on personal characteristics and levels of illness severity
➤ whether case managers would need to have the same or similar conditions as those they were working with, or whether any previous contact with mental health services would be beneficial
➤ what type of training and support would be required to ensure that service users and professionals felt confident in the provision
➤ whether providing additional training and support would make the service more or less cost effective than traditional services
➤ and what other added costs and benefits there might be, including to peer care managers themselves.

Unfortunately, the existing totality of evidence does not provide us with the answers to these questions, though most pilot studies and reviews conducted in the past 15 years have suggested the need to trial peer case managers more extensively. Is it time to consider setting up a pilot scheme in England?

If so, there are various conditions that may be needed to ensure safe and effective peer case management. Both the evidence review and feedback from service users and staff suggests that we would need readiness on the part of organisations and staff; staff training to readjust attitudes; training for service users; regular supervision; and adequate autonomy to 'do the job'. These principles are supported by broader reviews of involving clients in research and service development, both in the National Health Service (NHS) and internationally.[53] For example, one review concluded that 'productive methods for involving consumers require appropriate skills, resources and time to develop and follow appropriate working practices'.[54] The same is likely to be true for involving people with mental health needs as case managers for other service users. Time and organisational buy-in are both 'limited resources', and ones that would need to be in place in any pilot schemes in England.

Involvement of all relevant services may also be a potential success factor or barrier.

> 'I would like to see something like this tried out, but there are some real caveats. It would need to be properly resourced – and not just in terms of money, but also adequate training and supervision from professionals. And perhaps most importantly, there would need to be excellent communication, buy-in and leadership from all the services involved. The voluntary sector would need to know what was happening so we could provide support. Councils and home helps, health services, community mental health teams, families and service users – there would be lots of people to consult, inform, and engage with in any trial of this nature.'

> **Voluntary sector service provider from Newcastle**

Training is also an integral part of the process, not just for service users, but also for professionals themselves. There is evidence that professionals' attitudes can have an enormous impact on whether changes in policy and practice are successful.[55] One trial found that peer case managers were concerned about how they were perceived by professionals.[56] Therefore training professionals to accept and work alongside clients as professional colleagues may be important. Both US and UK studies have suggested that involving service users as trainers of mental health professionals can improve acceptance and result in more positive attitudes.[57,58] It would be interesting to see whether this would also hold in the field of peer case management.

This chapter does not suggest any solutions – but it does pose a number of questions to be answered in the continuing development of mental health services in England. In conclusion, it appears that there is mixed evidence and support for clients as professional colleagues in England, and many questions remain unanswered. But in focusing on person-centred care and in considering aspects of the path to recovery, do we owe it to our clients, our colleagues, and our communities to investigate further? The service users we spoke to certainly thought so.

> 'I was diagnosed with depression around the age of 16. I have been on dozens of anti-depressants, had so much therapy, and been hospitalised four times. At first I didn't want anyone to know. But then I got involved in helping others

and that's made a real difference to me, and hopefully to the people I support. I'm now working at a charity supporting others with depression and while I can't say it's all plain sailing, I do think that having someone to talk to that really knows what you're going through and has been there themselves makes a difference. I help find services to meet other people's needs and talk through issues. I like to think I complement professional services and add something unique. I think other people should have a chance to help others and to receive help from someone who really knows what its like.'

28-year-old Helene from Birmingham

REFERENCES

1 Elliot DL, Goldberg L, Moe EL, *et al*. Preventing substance use and disordered eating: initial outcomes of the ATHENA (athletes targeting healthy exercise and nutrition alternatives) program. *Arch Pediatr Adolesc Med*. 2004; **158**(11): 1043–9.

2 Randall BP, Eggert LL, Pike KC. Immediate post intervention effects of two brief youth suicide prevention interventions. *Suicide Life Threat Behav*. 2001; **31**(1): 41–61.

3 Cuijpers P. Peer-led and adult-led school drug prevention: a meta-analytic comparison. *J Drug Educ*. 2002; **32**(2): 107–19.

4 McAuliffe WE. A randomized controlled trial of recovery training and self-help for opioid addicts in New England and Hong Kong. *J Psychoactive Drugs*. 1990; **22**(2): 197–209.

5 Dennis CL. The effect of peer support on postpartum depression: a pilot randomized controlled trial. *Can J Psychiatry*. 2003; **48**(2): 115–24.

6 Bjorklund RW. Linking discharged patients with peers in the community. *Psychiatry Services*. 2000; **51**(10): 1316.

7 Kane CF, Blank MB. NPACT: enhancing programs of assertive community treatment for the seriously mentally ill. *Community Ment Health J*. 2004, **40**(6): 549–59.

8 Solomon P, Draine J. Consumer case management and attitudes concerning family relations among persons with mental illness. *Psychiatr Q*. 1995; **66**(3): 249–61.

9 Bettencourt T, Hodgins A, Huba GJ, *et al*. Bay Area Young Positives: a model of a youth-based approach to HIV/AIDS services. *J Adolesc Health*. 1998; **23**(2 Suppl): 28–36.

10 Forchuk C, Martin ML, Chan YL, *et al*. Therapeutic relationships: from psychiatric hospital to community. *J Psychiatr Ment Health Nurs*. 2005; **12**(5): 556–64.

11 Lyons JS, Cook JA, Ruth AR, *et al*. Service delivery using consumer staff in a mobile crisis assessment program. *Community Ment Health J*. 1996; **32**(1): 33–40.

12 Klein AR, Cnaan RA, Whitecraft J. Significance of peer support with dually diagnosed clients: findings from a pilot study. *Res Soc Work Pract*. 1998; **8**: 529–51.

13 Chien WT, Chan SW. One-year follow-up of a multiple-family-group intervention for Chinese families of patients with schizophrenia. *Psychiatr Serv*. 2004; **55**(11): 1276–84.

14 Kelly JA, McAuliffe TL, Sikkema KJ, *et al*. Reduction in risk behavior among adults with severe mental illness who learned to advocate for HIV prevention. *Psychiatr Serv*. 1997; **48**(10): 1283–8.

15 Mental Health Task Force User Group. *Forging Our Futures: lighting the fire.* London: Department of Health; 1995.

16 NHS Health Advisory Service. *Voices in Partnership: involving users and carers in commissioning and delivering mental health services.* London: HMSO; 1997.

17 Department of Health. *National Service Framework for Mental Health: modern standards and service models.* London: Department of Health; 1999.

18 *Case Management Competences Framework for the Care of People with Long Term Conditions.* London: NHS Modernisation Agency; Skills for Health; 2005.

19 Grech E. Case management: a critical analysis of the literature. *Int J Psychosocial Rehab.* 2002; **6**: 89–98.

20 Marshall M, Gray A, Lockwood A, *et al.* Case management for people with severe mental disorders. *Cochrane Database Syst Rev.* 2000; **2**: CD000050.

21 Albrecht GL, Peters KE. Peer intervention in case management practice. *J Case Manag.* 1997; **6**(2): 43–50.

22 Bedell JR, Cohen NL, Sullivan A. Case management: the current best practices and the next generation of innovation. *Community Ment Health J.* 2000; **36**(2): 1979–94.

23 Solomon P, Draine J. Satisfaction with mental health treatment in a randomized trial of consumer case management. *J Nerv Ment Dis.* 1994; **182**(3): 179–84.

24 Simpson EL, House AO. Involving users in the delivery and evaluation of mental health services: systematic review. *BMJ.* 2002; **325**: 1265.

25 Rodney M, Clasen C, Goldman G, *et al.* Three evaluation methods of a community health advocate program. *J Community Health.* 1998; **23**(5): 371–81.

26 Solomon P, Draine J. The efficacy of a consumer case management team: 2-year outcomes of a randomized trial. *J Ment Health Adm.* 1995; **22**(2): 135–46.

27 Chinman MJ, Rosenheck R, Lam JA, *et al.* Comparing consumer and non-consumer provided case management services for homeless persons with serious mental illness. *J Nerv Ment Dis.* 2000; **188**(7): 446–53.

28 Davidson L, Chinman M, Sells D, *et al.* Peer support among adults with serious mental illness: a report from the field. *Schizophr Bull.* 2006; **32**(3): 443–50.

29 Nyamathi A, Flaskerud JH, Leake B, *et al.* Evaluating the impact of peer, nurse case-managed, and standard HIV risk-reduction programs on psychosocial and health-promoting behavioral outcomes among homeless women. *Res Nurs Health.* 2001; **24**(5): 410–22.

30 Solomon P, Draine J, Delaney MA. The working alliance and consumer case management. *J Ment Health Adm.* 1995; **22**(2): 126–34.

31 Paulson R, Herinckx H, Demmler J, *et al.* Comparing practice patterns of consumer and non-consumer mental health service providers. *Community Ment Health J.* 1999; **35**(3): 251–69.

32 den Boer PC, Wiersma D, Russo S, *et al.* Paraprofessionals for anxiety and depressive disorders. *Cochrane Database Syst Rev.* 2005; **18**(2): CD004688.

33 Sells D, Davidson L, Jewell C, *et al.* The treatment relationship in peer-based and regular case management for clients with severe mental illness. *Psychiatr Serv.* 2006; **57**(8): 1179–84.

34 Clark CC, Scott EA, Boydell KM, *et al.* Effects of client interviewers on client-reported satisfaction with mental health services. *Psychiatr Serv.* 1999; **50**(7): 961–3.

35 Polowczyk D, Brutus M, Orvieto AA, *et al.* Comparison of patient and staff surveys of consumer satisfaction. *Hosp Community Psychiatry.* 1993; **44**: 589–91.

36 Felton CJ, Stastny P, Shern DL, *et al*. Consumers as peer specialists on intensive case management teams: impact on client outcomes. *Psychiatr Serv*. 1995; **46**(10): 1037–44.

37 O'Donnell M, Parker G, Proberts M, *et al*. A study of client-focused case management and consumer advocacy: the community and consumer service project. *Aust NZ J Psychiatry*. 1999; **33**: 684–93.

38 Solomon P, Draine J. Family perceptions of consumers as case managers. *Community Ment Health J*. 1994; **30**(2): 165–76.

39 Rodney M, Clasen C, Goldman G, *et al*. Three evaluation methods of a community health advocate program. *J Community Health*. 1998; **23**(5): 371–81.

40 Simon PM, Morse EV, Speier T, *et al*. Training older adults to work as psychiatric case management aides. *Hosp Community Psychiatry*. 1993; **44**(12): 1162–5.

41 Weissman EM, Covell NH, Kushner M, *et al*. Implementing peer-assisted case management to help homeless veterans with mental illness transition to independent housing. *Community Ment Health J*. 2005; **41**(3): 267–76.

42 Dixon L, Hackman A, Lehman A. Consumers as staff in assertive community treatment programs. *Adm Policy Ment Health*. 1997; **25**(2): 199–208.

43 Mowbray CT, Moxley DP, Thrasher S, *et al*. Consumers as community support providers: issues created by role innovation. *Community Ment Health J*. 1996; **32**(1): 47–67.

44 Meehan T, Bergen H, Coveney C, *et al*. Development and evaluation of a training program in peer support for former consumers. *Int J Ment Health Nurs*. 2002; **11**(1): 34–9.

45 Carlson LS, Rapp CA, McDiarmid D. Hiring consumer-providers: barriers and alternative solutions. *Community Mental Health J*. 2001; **37**(3): 199–213.

46 Ratzlaff S, McDiarmid D, Marty D, *et al*. The Kansas Consumer as Provider program: measuring the effects of a supported education initiative. *Psychiatr Rehab J*. 2006; **29**(3): 174–82.

47 McDiarmid D, Rapp C, Ratzlaff S. Design and initial results from a supported education initiative: the Kansas Consumer as Provider Program. *Psychiatric Rehab J*. 2005; **29**(1): 3–9.

48 Mowbray CT, Moxley DP, Collins ME. Consumers as mental health providers: first-person accounts of benefits and limitations. *J Behav Health Serv Res*. 1998; **25**(4): 397–411.

49 Solomon P, Draine J. Perspectives concerning consumers as case managers. *Community Ment Health J*. 1996; **32**(1): 41–6.

50 White H, Whelan C, Barnes JD, *et al*. Survey of consumer and non-consumer mental health service providers on assertive community treatment teams in Ontario. *Community Ment Health J*. 2003; **39**(3): 265–76.

51 Sherman PS, Porter R. Mental health consumers as case management aides. *Hosp Community Psychiatry*. 1991; **42**(5): 494–8.

52 Davidson L, Chinman M, Sells D, *et al*. Peer support among adults with serious mental illness: a report from the field. *Schizophr Bull*. 2006; **32**(3): 443–50.

53 Dixon L, Krauss N, Lehman A. Consumers as service providers: the promise and challenge. *Community Ment Health J*. 1994; **30**(6): 615–25.

54 Oliver S, Clarke-Jones L, Rees R, *et al*. Involving consumers in research and development agenda setting for the NHS: developing an evidence-based approach. *Health Technol Assess*. 2004; **8**(15): 1–148.

55 Singh D. *Making the Shift: key success factors.* Birmingham: University of Birmingham and NHS Centre for Innovation and Improvement; 2006.

56 Solomon P, Draine J. Perspectives concerning consumers as case managers. *Community Ment Health J.* 1996; **32**(1): 41–6.

57 Cook JA, Jonikas JA, Razzano L. A randomised evaluation of consumer versus non-consumer training of state mental health service providers. *Community Ment Health J.* 1995; **31**(3): 229–38.

58 Wood J, Wilson-Barnett J. The influence of user involvement on the learning of mental health nursing students. *NT Research.* 1999; **4**: 257–70.

CHAPTER 10

A personal account: from my life

ANDREW ROGERS

A moving and subtle description of being a user of services and of the pressures and opportunities encountered in a long – and continuing – journey through serious illness.

INTRODUCTION

This account is based on my experience in various hospital settings in England and Scotland since I was first diagnosed with schizophrenia whilst at university.

ADMISSION

'Would you like to go into hospital for a rest?' . . . and here I am, not in a general hospital at all, but at the frontier posts of the health services, an antique mental institution.

A stressed disorder rules on entry – patients milling around (some in dressing-gowns), staff observing, admissions procedures being followed just out of earshot, eventually some pills may be offered, and (if you are together enough) you may talk to some other residents over the near-obligatory cigarette. In this case though, after pacing around in a rather confused manner, I retire to the room and sleep intervenes.

A slight feeling of normality returns on entry to the dining-room with its associations with school or company canteen. Some residents may have eating disorders or anorexia, and so may not feel inclined to join in, though the staff may encourage them to take enough nutrition. If reliable sedatives or anti-psychotics have been issued, the patient may enter a more relaxed stage, maybe by the following evening. The sight of people relaxing in the lounge may induce at best the feeling of a family.

My first experience of mental health services was in the 1990s – well before *Big Brother*, but the lounge at a mental institution can present the better side of that scenario: community and involvement, but with a less competitive edge. In both cases it is a question of human dynamics, with varying results, from rough to smooth.

On my first admission, we wrote out the Leonard Cohen song *Anthem* ('Every heart to love will come, but like a refugee'), which at the time seemed to turn the whole operation into an exercise in righteous rebellion, making a stand for passion and solidarity, far opposed to the lone meanderings of the mind that occur in the dormitory. These feelings can arise because of the ever-present temptation to regard oneself as a victim or hostage to the health system. After discharge, the experience can be regarded in a more sober light with a correspondingly more positive view of the mental health system, but this is harder during the time of admission.

An acquaintance with another resident – a businessman with a wide knowledge of life gained from listening to Radio 4 – was the first indication that the experience would not be the straitjacketed mumbling inmate scenario one had expected from films. Instead there was rational if at times manic conversation, as each patient searched for their thought-orbit.

DIAGNOSIS

At first the diagnosis I was given was that 'You are experiencing problems with your mental health'. Later a short explanation of schizophrenia or manic depression might be attempted, though the patient is necessarily left to come to terms with the situation internally, and this can be an experience of fear and confusion, despite the often genuinely warm and helpful attention of the staff overseeing the admission.

Once this stage is passed, the patient's mental state may have calmed, to be replaced by another anxiety – the feeling of being a captive or 'inmate', rather than the more positive view that one is being secluded for one's welfare and greatest benefit.

Initially the search for company may lead the newly admitted resident to attempt to socialise with the other patients. This may work, but can also compound the mental confusion by association with equally disturbed minds. At this point there may resurface a strategy learned in childhood – a simple desire to be with 'adults' (the search for stability that Freud identified as the 'superego'), which leads the patient to stand or sit near the staff area, perhaps asking questions and feeling the protection and security that prevail in a family when the child is being 'good'.

And so the critical early stages of the admission pass, and a rhythm reasserts itself: visiting the dining-room, perhaps attending an 'OT' (occupational therapy) meeting, and socialising (or, at worst, chain-smoking) in the lounge. On my first admission we played croquet, and this seemed to create a more relaxed and friendly atmosphere, and though some patients would remain enigmatic or unapproachable, there were always enough fellow travellers to allow for some mentally stimulating conversation and emotional support.

Once the diagnosis had been made, I consulted a textbook to learn what 'schizophrenia' was, and found that the illness crystalised into two aspects: the simple medical explanation was that an excessive amount of the neurotransmitter dopamine was causing unstable brain activity, leaving the mind over-stimulated and unbalanced. The second side of the issue was social/existential: the affected person may find it difficult to fit into society or achieve a normal life pattern. The psychosis was often accompanied by alienation and a downward spiral in social terms, though there was an opposite pole – the triumph of human imagination and will portrayed in the film *A Beautiful Mind*. This offered the consoling idea that, even if one was suffering from mental ill-health, one could be a genius in the same category as Vincent Van Gogh or Sylvia Plath. This perspective is confirmed by reading *Voices*, the magazine of the National Schizophrenia Fellowship.

'ESCAPE'

But always in a confined situation such as a mental hospital, whether one dislikes or covertly enjoys the experience, there lurks the perennial theme of 'escape'. The more stable patients may be committed to seeing the process through to the date of discharge suggested by the consultant. The less stable, or simply wilder, people may be entertaining thoughts of 'breaking out' and setting off back home or simply out into the wilds.

If the patient is able to relax and trust in the process of his or her recuperation, the experience can be a positive one. You are freed from the necessity of earning a living, or studying for an exam, and can simply make the best of the surrounding environment, and the intriguing characters one may not have run into in the course of everyday life. For example, on my first admission I met a laboratory assistant with some unusual ideas of scientists replacing politicians as the arbiters of society. Such conversations, like the inevitable positive thinking/self-help manuals found in these scenarios, can be a liberating introduction to wider horizons of thought and inspirations.

Once the seriousness of the condition is apprehended, the patient may be thrown back on his or her resources for perhaps the first time in a long while; and though this may be disorienting at first, it can also allow the mind to seek new directions and develop new psychological strategies, releasing dormant faculties in a potentially positive and constructive way. Such a scenario – people gently discussing ideas over a cigarette, while intelligently assessing their pharmaceutical requirements – is at the more positive pole of the spectrum.

On other occasions, one may be doped up on medication, surrounded by unfamiliar or unsympathetic people, while the television brashly emits constant noise. In these situations the desire to 'go over the wall' may be overwhelming, and one may be continually on the look-out for opportunities to break out of the ward. Once out there, however, the world can be forbidding – perhaps a row of suburban streets or even expansive countryside may greet the exploring patient with the lonely challenge of wandering without resources, money or direction. The reaction to this may be to turn back to the ward, now perceived as a nurturing sanctuary and shelter from reality. Hopefully the patient/escapee may value the services offered more highly and embrace the therapeutic routine until a more appropriate and officially agreed time of discharge.

PROGRESS

So much, however, is dependent on the people encountered. If they are sympathetic, the experience will be potentially positive; if not, you can only retire with a book or Walkman – people need people.

And so events take their course and (in a best-case scenario) the patient receives the information and medication he or she needs, and sets forth from the institution armed with a better self-knowledge, a stronger support network, and perhaps most importantly some new mental strategies to guide him or her along the upcoming journey. In a less successful situation the patient may feel resentful, or simply not understand the rationale behind the diagnosis. In this case, the required compliance with medication may be avoided, and a cycle of re-admissions becomes likely. The time and resources needed for each new admission make it highly desirable that the newly discharged patient maintains a good level of progress and a strong inner constitution.

In conclusion, I would like to observe that, while medication may be an essential part of recovery from mental illness, we perhaps overstress the categorical distinction between the mentally 'healthy' and 'unhealthy'.

Schizophrenia is regarded as a psychosis, but the dictionary defines it simply as 'a disharmony in thoughts, feelings and actions'. It is this human disharmony that both Eastern ('Right-Mindfulness') and Western ('Integration') psycho-therapeutic approaches seek to cure. From this view point, mental health service users (though needing a special approach) can be seen as one tributary of the common ethical and moral river of humanity.

CHAPTER 11

Working with young people: 24 hours in the life of The Highfield Family and Adolescent Unit, Oxford

FRANCIS JOSEPHS

The account of the work of The Highfield which follows is written largely from my own perspective (educational, then nursing), and therefore one which other colleagues might view differently. I was appointed in 1990 from a teaching background, having been Head of English and then Head of Sixth at a comprehensive in Oxford. After six years I became teacher in charge of the school in the Unit, and took early retirement in 2003, staying on as a part-time teacher until 2005. I then left, but quickly realised how much I missed the environment. So I returned a few months later to take up a post with the nursing team as a care assistant three days a week, a post I find both fascinating and very rewarding.

INTRODUCTION

The Highfield Family and Adolescent Unit is located in a very pleasant environment in Headington, Oxford, in the leafy, Victorian grounds of The Warneford Hospital. The Unit caters for adolescents with acute psychiatric disorders, admitting young people up to the age of 18 primarily from Oxfordshire and Buckinghamshire, as well as from Northamptonshire, Berkshire and surrounding counties. The Unit, which is part of the Oxfordshire and Buckinghamshire Mental Health Partnership Trust, employs a short to medium length of stay policy. Most of our patients are aged 13–17, though we are currently planning to admit 11- and 12-year-olds; the majority are voluntary patients, though some are admitted on a section of the Mental Health Act.

We have 14 inpatient beds, and can also take up to four day-patients. We are not a secure unit, though we do have a seclusion room; patients who require a short period of extra containment as part of their treatment may be transferred to the Intensive Care Unit in the main hospital, if this is deemed suitable. The Highfield includes single and dormitory accommodation, social areas including a lounge, kitchen, games room and private garden, as well as offices, meeting rooms and a school. The Unit was set up in 1972; since 1988 Dr Anthony James has been the consultant in charge. There is a separate outpatient service but this chapter focuses solely on my area of experience, which is the inpatient work.

We accept both routine and emergency medical referrals, and admit patients with a wide range of acute conditions. These include individuals with eating disorders, psychoses, obsessive-compulsive disorders, depression, anxiety disorders, borderline personality, bipolar disorder, attention deficit hyperactive disorder (ADHD), post-traumatic stress disorder (PTSD) and deliberate self-harm. In addition we admit patients with autistic spectrum disorder, conduct disorder, drug and alcohol problems, chronic fatigue, or with mild to moderate learning disabilities – *provided* that there is evidence that they also have a serious psychiatric condition. We offer a range of treatment programmes, tailored to the individual's needs and developmental status, including psychological, behavioural, cognitive, group and family therapies. Pharmacotherapy is also used, for instance, in the treatment of psychotic and major affective disorders. We employ a multi-disciplinary model of working, which has immense advantages but can also be very time-consuming and difficult to get right. Staff from a wide range of disciplines work together to provide and develop tailor-made care plans and programmes for every patient. Apart from the nurses, care assistants and doctors, the disciplines include teachers, occupational therapists, psychologists, social workers, dieticians, counsellors and pharmacists. The Unit is also a training placement for students from many of these disciplines, and it is fascinating to hear them say how worried many were about this particular placement. The majority viewed with great concern the prospect of the 'double-whammy' of working not only with the mentally ill but also with those 'dreaded' teenagers. In reality they often discover that many days at Highfield are delightful, full of laughter, pleasant banter and rewarding progress; a minority can be stressful and challenging.

Every day at Highfield is very different indeed, which is precisely part of its attraction, whilst at the same time a source of potential problems. However, the best way of conveying what we do, and of offering a flavour of the atmosphere, is to attempt to describe a typical day. The outline timetable below includes some of what is on offer.

HIGHFIELD SCHOOL – PUPIL TIMETABLE – pupils of school age to attend for all sessions

DAY	9.30–9.45	10.00–11.00	11.00–11.20	11.20–12.15	12.15–1.30	1.30–2.30	2.30–3.30	3.45
Monday	Morning meeting	Assembly Key teacher time	BREAK		LUNCH		Physical education/games Unit activity – to include all young people	Highfield Unit Group (HUG) Meeting
Tuesday	Morning meeting	Play reading option	BREAK	Pottery option	LUNCH	Personal, social, health and citizenship education Unit (PSHCE) activity – to include all young people	Activities Unit activity – to include all young people	Afternoon meeting
Wednesday	9.00 Ward review	10.45 Morning meeting	BREAK	Environment group or 16+ group	LUNCH	Plan cooking		Afternoon meeting
Thursday	Morning meeting	Drama group option	BREAK		LUNCH	Art group Unit activity – to include all young people		Afternoon meeting
Friday	Morning meeting	Key teacher time	BREAK	Key teacher time	LUNCH	Afternoon trip – to include all young people		Afternoon meeting

EARLY MORNING

At about 7.15 a.m. the night-staff welcomes the early shift with a cup of tea and a detailed handover of the previous ten hours' events. Patients are awoken at around 8.00 a.m. (not the easiest of jobs with teenagers!), medicines administered, weights noted and observations checked. A minority of patients will be on level 2 or level 3 observations, when there are significant concerns for their safety, or that of others. These are constantly reviewed, as we are reluctant to continue them for longer than is absolutely necessary: patients can become dependent on them and/or or resent them, and they impose heavy demands on staffing. From a staff point of view, they are tricky to carry out. You have to avoid being over-intrusive, whilst at the same time ensuring safety. You need to remain positive and supportive, whilst also avoiding rewarding bad behaviour/habits with attention. Long periods of level 3 do make great demands on staff, and morale is lowered after long periods of shifts which seem to consist of nothing but observations, with little scope for more creative work.

Restraint is another area which can cause staff difficulty. We employ a wide range of techniques and strategies to ensure that any potentially difficult situation is avoided or defused. However, very occasionally an individual's behaviour escalates to such an extent that their safety, or that of other staff or young people, is endangered. In these circumstances, after formal warnings, restraint is undertaken. Although staff are rigorously trained for such eventualities, it is a procedure which can be distressing, not only for the patient themselves but for the staff involved. This is usually followed by isolation to a purpose-built safe area. Such isolation is seen as very short-term – a matter of a few hours at the very most, with the emphasis on the individual's return to the ward, initially on level 3 observations. In extreme circumstances we might consider a brief transfer to the secure adult Intensive Care Unit, which is nearby on the site, with regular daily visits from our staff. Our aim would be to return them to our Unit within a few days; very occasionally this proves impossible, and we then have to consider a transfer to a secure adolescent unit elsewhere. In my experience, I would estimate that this latter eventuality might happen once every two years or so.

To return to early morning routines, once these are completed, breakfast is then prepared. This (and all meal preparations) is a tricky job, as those with eating disorders each have subtly different and ever-changing diet plans which need to be adhered to precisely. All meals at Highfield are seen as an integral part of the treatment for all patients, and it is viewed as important that everyone attends to the end, and then helps with clearing and laying the table for the next meal. The role of staff at such times requires great skill, as they need to maintain a normal 'family' atmosphere, whilst at the same time ensuring that some individuals eat the minimum required, and that others, especially those on certain medications, do not over-eat. Not an easy task!

9.00 A.M.

It is now 9.00 and some young people have free time, though others on eating programmes are supervised in the lounge. At the same time, the nurses provide a 30-minute handover for the multi-disciplinary staff. On Wednesdays, this is replaced by a two-hour ward review, at which all staff discuss each patient in turn, and make plans for the future. This is seen as one of the most important meetings of the week, and very often real differences of emphasis emerge, creative sparks fly and important decisions are made which enable each patient to move forward, or to cope with a difficult stage of their treatment. I have always been very impressed by the prevalent culture which enables the most junior member of the team to have their say, receive an honest feedback and to influence the argument. (I have to admit that there was a period, some 10 years ago or so, when this was not always the case, and staff relationships were sometimes adversely affected, with damaging splits developing.) Decisions are now arrived at with great care, taking into account the needs and views of the young person and of his or her family, whilst at the same time focusing on considerations of safety. When, for example, observations are lessened, a diet plan is changed, leave is increased, or 10-minute walks alone in the grounds are introduced, we realise we are taking a calculated risk in order to move forward. I firmly believe that this is now one of the current strengths of the Unit: that we are able to come to a group decision after careful thought, and support each other if the consequences are not always those we hoped for. I remember some years ago racking my brains as a new teacher on the Unit, trying to engage a deeply unwell 16-year-old girl who sat in a depressed silence, unable/unwilling to participate in any activity whatsoever. One day I eventually noticed her staring at a Van Gogh poster, gave her some paints and left her. When I returned she had tentatively begun to copy it, and this gradually led to more creative work, culminating in a written project on the artist. The nurses immediately noticed how much better she interacted, both in and out of school, and I received lots of pleasing feedback. I basked in this achievement until one day the charge nurse took me aside and told me that the girl had attempted during the night, like Vincent in the past, to cut her earlobe off. I was devastated and very worried; he, however, reassured me that the benefits to her had hugely outweighed the minor setback, and the team was very supportive to me personally. The girl did continue to improve, and was discharged before long (with a healed earlobe); she later told me she got an 'A' on her GCSE art Van Gogh project!

At 9.30 on other days the morning meeting takes place, which is attended by all patients and as many staff on duty as possible. It is seen as a vital part of the treatment, offering an opportunity for anyone to raise any issue, and see it discussed, as well as setting the scene for the day, and welcoming anyone new – or saying goodbye. The young people are encouraged to chair the meeting in turn, which has a fixed agenda: 'Meeting open; Apologies; Announcements; Nurses on duty; Meetings; Negatives; Positives; Any other business'. The meetings vary considerably: they can be short and routine, amusing, very stressful, argumentative, nostalgic, bitter, dull, uplifting –sometimes all of these!

10.00 A.M.

The school bell rings at 10.00 a.m., and all younger pupils have to attend full-time every day. Those beyond the school-leaving age must attend all Unit activities (run in conjunction with the occupational therapists (OTs)), which amount to half the timetable. They can then choose to opt into other sessions, depending on their interests and motivation. Some pupils queue to go up to school; some are reluctant for a range of personal, medical and behavioural reasons. There are sometimes frustrating periods when a small group consistently refuse to attend Unit structures. However, it is undeniable that over the years the school has had a consistent record of educational and social success with the majority of patients, including some who for years had found mainstream school difficult, for a multitude of reasons. Each pupil has a key teacher, who is part of the multi-disciplinary case team, and who ensures that an appropriate curriculum is delivered; he or she liaises with the pupil's own school, ensuring that relevant coursework is obtained, and that reintegration takes place if and when the time is right. Some pupils will go on extended leave prior to discharge, or be given support in visiting their school or possibly a new establishment. Pupils sit public examinations at Highfield if necessary. During the school holidays, OTs take a lead with nurses in ensuring that a stimulating programme of activities continues. OTs also have primary responsibility for the timetable of those aged 16 and over, beyond the school-leaving age.

LATE MORNING

After a morning break, school resumes until 12.15 p.m. During the school day many other activities are taking place: patients sometimes have to miss a school session in order to attend a family meeting, case team meeting or care programme approach (CPA) meeting; or an individual session with their primary nurse, OT, link worker, doctor, key teacher, psychologist, physiotherapist, outreach worker, connexions officer, outreach worker or other professional. All of these meetings are seen as a crucial part of every patient's treatment, and important issues are discussed in depth, feelings explored, advice given and short- and long-term plans made and regularly fine-tuned – or sometimes radically reassessed! Young people (and their parents) often find the family meetings the most difficult part of their treatment on the Unit, and attendance at these is an essential commitment made at admission. Very difficult issues are explored, often for the first time, and raw emotions exposed. I remember being involved in my first such meeting many years ago, and feeling very shattered by the intense interactions I had witnessed. Dr James, however, seemed very positive and calm, pointing out to me that the family had at last begun to address the relevant issues, and that progress would now surely follow. Interestingly, families seem to find multi-family therapy a more positive experience. Several families are brought together for three days to discuss their experiences, and to share problems and solutions with staff and each other.

Another crucial meeting which takes place every four weeks or so is the CPA meeting. The link worker arranges meetings of all staff involved in the care of the young person, together with their family and with relevant outside agencies. The first half consists of reports from all concerned, and the second of plans for the future. Difficult but vital issues are discussed: How are things going at home and on the Unit? What changes in treatment, groups, medication, leave, care plans, school attendance and so on need to be made? It is an opportunity for compliments and criticism, and strong opinions and feelings do often emerge. Not surprisingly, the CPA is occasionally seen to be a vehicle for young people (and sometimes for their parents) to blame the Unit very forcefully for all their problems. This can be very hard for staff, who have worked tirelessly and patiently, to hear. At such times it is vital for staff to get the right balance: on the one hand not to agonise over patently unfair charges, whilst at the same time being prepared to accept that the outburst might reveal shortcomings on our part, which need to be rectified.

During the day many other professional and management meetings take place. The nurses meet daily, sometimes with the consultant, sometimes with the dietician. Multi-disciplinary weekly meetings with psychotherapists take place, so that individual and group issues can be explored in depth. All staff have regular individual supervision, as well as access to a weekly 50-minute 'Reflections' slot, with an outside facilitator. Both provide an invaluable opportunity to explore and assess difficult issues, and to find creative solutions to problems and areas of stress. There is also a wide range of teaching sessions throughout the day, both within disciplines, and of a multi-disciplinary nature. In addition, on many days staff are engaged in assessing a possible referral to the Unit, and making the decision as to whether we are able to help, or whether a further period of outpatient support would be better. Sometimes we have to put an admission on hold, as we are often full, with a waiting list. The actual process of admission is a necessarily lengthy and comprehensive process. We realise how nervous (or indeed resistant) the young person and their family are likely to be, and we do our best to reassure and orientate them fully. We ensure the individual becomes aware both of their rights, and of the Unit's expectations. She or he is introduced to their link worker and primary nurse, senior members of staff who will coordinate the work of their case team and ensure that a care plan is created and that regular CPA meetings take place.

THE AFTERNOON

Lunch takes place at 12.30 p.m., with afternoon school resuming at 1.30 p.m. By now the afternoon shift staff are beginning to take over from their weary 'early' colleagues. The priority in such transitions is to ensure that a clear handover takes place – we are all aware of the risk of communication problems inherent in the shift system, and some of our patients are very quick to exploit any ambiguities or omissions! The afternoon school slots tend to be mainly group sessions, sometimes taking place off the Unit. These include physical education, swimming, climbing, art group and the Friday trip. We have exclusive access to a gym, a pool and a wall for the first three activities, and our own minibus for trips. The venues for the trip vary extensively, including museums and University, parks, countryside and canals, ice-rinks and bowling complexes. Once a term, and in holidays, we organise more extended trips to venues further afield, such as wildlife parks, London, the coast or the rainforest (at Newbury rather than Costa Rica). All such activities are seen as very important and beneficial in improving self-confidence, and avoiding institutionalisation. For many young people, however, trips raise difficult issues of past experiences, obsessions or fear of the outside world, and they need careful persuasion. Staff are also juggling with complex factors: have Section 17s been signed? Has parental approval been received? Does the person's activity level/care plan permit this activity? Are extra staff needed? What medication needs to be on hand? For all these reasons and more, trips off the Unit can be stressful for staff as well as for some patients.

At 3.45 p.m. the afternoon meeting takes place, a less structured community meeting to enable staff and patients to mull over the day. On Mondays, however, a longer 45-minute meeting occurs – the Highfield Unit Group (HUG). This is facilitated by a small group of staff, and it enables patients to address in depth issues relating to their feelings, thoughts and relationships. It can be a painful and raw occasion, but often a fruitful and rewarding session with new insights gained by patients and staff alike.

4.00 P.M.

The 4.00 p.m. tea break is often the time at which young people's birthdays and departures are marked with cards and cakes, a very important ritual of Highfield life. It also marks the end of the more structured part of the day, as the majority of the non-nursing staff begin to leave. Young people are given more periods of free time, and a greater degree of responsibility and choice. Some choose to socialise or to read or study, or to go for a walk, if their care plan allows. Some will watch television or play pool or table-tennis. Some will be phoning or texting or just thinking through difficult issues alone; some will be seeking help. This is clearly an essential and valuable period, but one fraught with problems for staff. Whilst many patients use the time in the positive ways outlined above, others take the opportunity to engage in less desirable activities. Some might choose to over-isolate themselves; some might abscond, some might self-harm. Self-harming, usually by cutting, is an increasing response to stress by some patients, and can be very distressing for all concerned. Staff are trained to be sympathetic and understanding, but also firm in their response. The emphasis is on trying to give lots of time to the patient who seeks out staff when they feel like self-harming, and to offer support and alternative strategies.

This late afternoon period is also one in which more meetings of the sort described earlier might be scheduled, as well as other post-school sessions. These currently include weekly basketball, physiotherapy and multi-gym sessions, dialectical behaviour therapy (DBT) or cognitive behavioural therapy (CBT) groups, the eating disorder group, an assertiveness group, and the Wednesday cooking group. In this latter group the young people, having chosen and budgeted their recipe, shop in the morning at the local Tescos, and then communally prepare and cook the meal in the afternoon. The session is sometimes fraught, but the results nearly always delicious.

EVENING AND OVERNIGHT

After the 6.00 p.m. meal, from 6.30 p.m. to 9.00 p.m., family and friends are free to visit, and the games room and garden are often lively with young people, parents, grandparents and young siblings. Those patients who are able to, will go out on leave for the evening, or overnight; others will leave the premises for an hour or two, with their family. Staff are constantly juggling with the endless permutations this throws up: some are desperate to go on leave, but it is deemed not appropriate yet, or their parents cannot/will not facilitate this. Others are unwilling, for a host of complicated and powerful reasons, to leave the Unit, and long negotiations/discussion/arguments can ensue. This period also offers an invaluable opportunity for staff to engage individuals in a more relaxed setting: over a pool table, on a stroll in the lovely South Parks opposite, or on a trip to the local shop. Evening drinks are at 9.30 p.m., by which time the night shift has taken over, and bed-time is at 11.00 p.m. This is always an unpredictable time with teenagers, but usually they retire cheerfully, after a certain amount of ritual posturing or grumbling. Occasionally things can get tricky, but are nearly always resolved by the traditional parental balancing act of tender loving care and Oscar-winning shows of firmness.

At 11.30 p.m. it's 'lights out' for the young people, but the start of a long night for the staff – a night of observations and rounds, and of innumerable administration tasks, culminating in the preparation of the breakfast table for the morning staff . . .

CONCLUSIONS, MEMORIES AND CREATIVE CONTRIBUTIONS

It's hard to know how to end this account of the workings of the Highfield Unit. Over the past 17 years I have found it a very inspiring and immensely rewarding place to work. I feel privileged not only to have worked with an incredibly talented, hard-working and dedicated team of staff, but also to have got to know so many remarkable and stimulating young people. I have lots of happy and funny memories, though inevitably there have also been some stressful and sad times too. Some young people were admitted highly distressed and very ill, often staying with us for long periods, sometimes with repeated admissions over several years. Many eventually left much more happy, able to return to their families, and better able to cope with the pressures of life. Sadly, some have not done as well, and to my knowledge, over the past 17 years, some four boys have taken their lives in the months/years after leaving us. However, on the positive side, quite a few have written moving accounts of their experiences here, either at the time, or from a distance of time. I would like to conclude this piece with two memories, selected from so very many.

The first is about a 15-year-old Somali refugee who arrived in a highly distressed, psychotic state on the Unit. He was initially very difficult to manage, and was often unreachable, in a world of his own. We eventually persuaded Khaleed (not his real name) to come up to school, but he would not engage at all. One day, in desperation, I played him a recording of Vivaldi's *The Four Seasons*, and gave him some paper and paints, to see if it would stimulate him at all. There was no reaction, so I left him to attend to another pupil in another room. This took longer than I had anticipated, so I hurried back to check he was alright. I entered the room to behold a moving sight: Khaleed was slowly dancing to the music in a wonderful, rhythmic manner, his steps precise, his hand movements echoing those of his feet, his face lit up by a glowing smile. It was the first of many little breakthroughs, and of a gradual improvement in his illness. This, of course did lead to a greater self-awareness on his part, and I remember his uncontrollable sobbing on his 16th birthday, as he speculated whether his whole life was to be thus. But my last memory of him was different. It was some four months on, and although he had improved he was still very afraid to face the future, and had consistently resisted our efforts to move him towards discharge. I was driving him back in my car from a swimming trip, one of those magical sunny March days, when for the first time for months you can smell summer and warmth in the air. I rolled my window down, and then he did alike with his, and by the time we got to the Unit, we had the sunroof up too. We sat in the car for a while saying nothing, and then he turned to me, and said, 'Time to go, Francis.'

I replied, 'Yes, we'll be late for the afternoon meeting.'

Khaleed turned to me, smiled, and said very calmly, 'No, you don't understand, Francis – it is time to go.' He began to work constructively towards his discharge, and was gone within two weeks, a confident and happy member of society.

The second memory is a more recent one, written by a lovely, highly talented girl who was first admitted when she was 13. She had a number of admissions over the next few years, some lengthy and some brief, but she always struggled valiantly with her problems, and was invariably warm and supportive towards peers and staff. She left us not long ago, very much better. As she was approaching the age of 18 she was aware that this was to be her last contact with us, and so she wrote the valedictory piece below:

HIGHFIELD

What a strange relationship we've had;
At times you've been a prison,

with metaphoric bars;
Being pinned down and restrained
has left me with mental scars.
At times you've been a sanctuary
when the world became too much,
picked me up, put me back on track,
got me back in touch.
Most people these days have no idea
what this sort of place is like,
they smile, laugh and giggle,
just at the prefix 'psych'.
They're 'nutjobs', they're 'wacko', they're 'loony',
the ones that live in there,
they hear things, see things, starve themselves,
then drown in their own despair.
People go by what they've seen in films,
or even on TV.
But if I had to stay in hospital,
then Highfield it would be:
with staff as good as them,
it would be easier being me.
They're kind, caring and willing,
always try their best,
so busy, in meetings here and there,
they never have time to rest.
Young people also play a part
in helping one another,
you end up feeling like they are
a sister or a brother.
The days are structured
with school, art group and PE,
and just when you think you've got a minute,
it's time for bloody tea!
I have memories both good and bad
of being here over the years.
Some I'd like to leave behind
with all my fallen tears;
Others I will hold on to
when things are getting tough.
For these, the words to thank Highfield

just never seem enough.
Thank you for having faith in me
when all my hope had gone.
You dragged me far away from death,
showed me how to carry on.
For Highfield I am thankful
for everything, it's true;
To all the doctors, nurses, teachers, OTs
I wouldn't be here today, if it wasn't for you.

Reproduced with permission.

CHAPTER 12

Creating a small community

TONY LINGIAH

This first-hand account by an experienced forensic nurse of creating a small nursing home emphasises the need for well-defined and articulated standards and visible leadership. It demonstrates that quality is not incompatible with commercial success.

INTRODUCTION

These pages tell a story. In many ways it is a simple one. It is told from the point of view of a long-standing aspiration, and embedded in care values and principles I have learnt from patients suffering from mental illness. In another sense, it is a story of the biggest risk taken, as failure would have been catastrophic for my family.

My career over the last forty years has given me the opportunity to work as a clinician, an educator and a manager – the whole spectrum of the healthcare arena, but the most profound impact on me as a professional and a person has been the relationships I developed with some psychiatric patients in institutions. Some of the experiences of service provision and staff attitudes spurred me on to a vision that I had secretly nurtured for a number of years . . . to create a small service which would treat people suffering from mental illness with humanity, warmth and compassion, and to create opportunities for them to reclaim their individuality and identity. This is the story of Abbeyfield Lodge.

THE BEGINNING

The vision was influenced by several factors, mainly derived from the proximity of my contact with people damaged by the distress of mental illness, and the frustration of not being able to do enough to alleviate their pain. Although I lacked entrepreneurial experience, I felt confident that my commitment and determination would play a key factor in realising my vision.

After several weeks of discussion and reflection, a business plan which was viable, credible and realistic was formulated and successfully submitted to the bank. We acquired a business which was already registered in the care sector, and converted it into a modern 12-bed home which was to be run on hotel principles underpinned by professional care.

THE SERVICE

Abbeyfield Lodge was registered as a care home for people with mental illness within the age range of 18–64 years, and subsequently changed to registered nursing home. The service provided a warm, friendly, comfortable and safe environment, staffed by registered mental nurses and healthcare assistants. The care team was supported by a business manager, clinical psychologist, activities coordinator, housekeeper, catering and support staff. The building dated back to the 1900s and was originally two separate adjoining houses in a terrace of three cottages, with the local post office forming the end terrace. The interior design and refurbishment helped to create a quality, homely environment, with very positive comments from residents and visitors.

Our aim was to create a small service where people who had been bruised by institutional experiences could start to reclaim their identity as individuals. The core principles underlying service provision were integrated in our philosophy of promoting respect, providing support and understanding and working with compassion to provide a service responsive to individual needs within a flexible framework. We also promoted the notion of freedom with responsibility, and the need for boundary setting and maintenance. We felt that this was an important element of community living. We provided comprehensive in-service training for all our staff to ensure that they were committed to our philosophy of care and service delivery. We also emphasised the concept that the team creates the ethos and if we could all demonstrate compassion and humanity, the service would acquire the hallmarks of a true quality service. Environmental cleanliness, respect for people, warm sympathetic approach, ability to anticipate needs became integrated in our daily routine.

It was important to be clear about the standard of service that was expected from staff, and equally, the standard of behaviour expected from residents. In practice, we found that team briefing, staff meetings and training sessions became essential tools of communication and feedback. Individual supervision sessions ensured that staff felt supported and understood. Regular meetings together for residents and staff helped to promote better understanding of working and living in a small community. This also provided a platform to discuss the week's events and activities and other in-house issues.

MANAGEMENT AND PRINCIPLES OF A GOOD SERVICE

The management of a mental health service and the frameworks under which it operates play a major part in achieving its central objective – to provide people with the care and attention they require to live happy, healthy and fulfilling lives.

For a service to be successful, its management must give attention to creating and maintaining the environment in which care takes place, to building up and sustaining the group of staff who will be the core people in delivering and supporting care, and to establishing a robust framework of quality checks which promote and enhance the service.

The aim must always be to promote a way of life for people, which permits them to enjoy, to the greatest extent possible, their rights as individual human beings. Therefore service delivery must be underpinned by some core principles. Abbeyfield Lodge established an ethos where respect, dignity and supportive care of the individual became the main threads of our daily interactions with people. These guiding principles incorporated the following themes: privacy, dignity, independence, civil rights and fulfilment.

PRIVACY

Each person had a comfortable en-suite bedroom with modern furniture and personal items to promote a sense of individuality. Most of the residents preferred to use housekeeping services and privacy was always respected prior to accessing individual rooms which were lockable. In the same way, confidentiality of information was always respected. The living space exceeded legislative requirements, so residents had access to several private areas during the day or night . . . where they felt secure, safe and in their personal space. We found that this reduced irritability and promoted an atmosphere of calmness and serenity.

DIGNITY

This is a complex but essential requirement of a good service. In practice, promoting the right to dignity involves recognising the intrinsic value of people's unique qualities as individuals and the specific nature of each resident's particular needs. Positive interactions, warm and supportive environments allowing people to express their views and participate in their care promote a sense of 'being in control'. Equally, de-stigmatising mental illness and working with compassion reduces the feelings of exclusion and helps in maintaining the dignity of the individual. Trusting relationships and a caring ethos give people confidence and enhances self-worth, so lacking in people who have been damaged by institutional experiences.

INDEPENDENCE

Institutions, by their nature, have to stick to routine and people are expected to fit in with little or no flexibility. Over a period of time, the institution eats into the very fabric of the person receiving care, and a sense of hopelessness and helplessness develops. Some symptoms of mental illness affect motivation and this further increases the sense of apathy in people. Gradually they become depersonalised, with a feeling of chronicity which requires great effort to reverse. Promoting independence prevents and reduces this state of dependency on the institution. Independence means having opportunities to think, act and make decisions – taking reasonable risks. Abbeyfield Lodge strove to provide people with discreet support and encouragement to stay in control of as many aspects of their lives as possible. We promoted a relationship based on trust, maturity and an attitude of exercising freedom with responsibility. Initially staff were concerned about allowing residents to take risks – such as going to the local shop on their own – and were anxious about incidents and gossips if something were to go wrong in the local community involving one of our residents. The principle that we would do everything possible to reduce risks and minimise danger, whilst at the same time acknowledging that we cannot guarantee a totally safe or risk-free lifestyle, gave everybody the confidence to manage situations on an individual needs basis.

CIVIL RIGHTS

Mental health problems are inextricably linked with civil rights issues. Compulsory detention in psychiatric institutions, albeit a necessity for a minority of people, is a complex process which requires a sensitive and robust framework. There is well-documented evidence that people suffering from mental health problems do experience discrimination and exclusion, thus restricting their ability to exercise their citizenship rights. It is therefore essential that services such as Abbeyfield Lodge provide a comprehensive framework which actively promotes opportunities for residents to access facilities and engage with the wider community, thus enabling them to achieve their full civil rights as citizens of a democracy. We ensured that all our residents were made aware of their right to vote.

FULFILMENT

One of the major implications of people's suffering from mental illness is their inability to maximise their potential, and this is not helped by the discriminatory attitude of people towards mental illness, especially in employment. Loss of friends, social contacts and income tend to restrict access to many sources of fulfilment. It is imperative that healthcare workers make attempts to compensate for these deprivations, by responding to individual needs and by creating opportunities for people to interact positively with the wider community in the spheres of work, leisure and education.

Abbeyfield Lodge incorporated into its philosophy the respect for rights and for needs of the individual, to enable them to take control of their lives, thus bringing hope, compassion, healing and humanity. Our service frameworks demonstrated a balance of care and responsibility, support and independence. Compassion and professionalism reflected in an environment which promoted and sustained a good quality of life for people in our care. We respected the need for medication, but exercised vigilance in its prescription and usage and our sector psychiatrist was very committed to regular reviews of both medication and care plans, thus reducing medication to the lowest safe level. We also encouraged informal discussion on the effects and side-effects of medication, thus creating a feeling of control and a sense of sharing in the management of medication.

WHAT CONCERNS DID WE HAVE?

Small businesses rely on maintaining maximum occupancy to ensure a consistent level of income. When a vacancy arose, it was crucial to plan for a new admission promptly. Referrals need to be followed up in a systematic way, and assessment organised to fit in with the timescale of the vacancy. Funding panels usually convened on a monthly basis – so delays could be costly to the service. We also experienced cash-flow problems, as first payments could only be effected when all administrative procedures were complete and approval obtained for payment. In some cases we waited several weeks before being included in the 'pay run', which can adversely affect a small business. On the whole, once a contract was set up, an automatic cycle of invoices and payments was effected. Our relationship with providers proved to be very satisfactory, based on establishing good communication channels.

CLINICAL ASSESSMENTS

A robust assessment protocol ensured that patients were thoroughly reviewed for suitability for placement at Abbeyfield Lodge. A mix of residents in whom there were areas of conflict would impact on interactions and would affect the way the services were delivered. Patients with a history of aggression and violence, personality disorder, drug and alcohol misuse, need to be managed by skilled staff who are able to set and maintain boundaries. Our greatest problems were those from individuals who had a history of arson and who threatened to use fire-setting as a behavioural tactic. They created a sense of insecurity and unease among staff and required strict fire protocols and staff vigilance. We found that on some occasions, this rigid framework impacted on our therapeutic milieu.

STAFF ISSUES

Small residential businesses depend on a staff team who work collaboratively to deliver a demanding service. The dynamics of relationships in a small staff team can create personality clashes and conflicts, which can damage the quality of the service. Our experience in the early months required us to work very hard to create harmony in the staff team and strong leadership ensured that problems were explored and managed in a mature and sensitive way. Some staff relationship problems, however, were more difficult to manage than patients' pathologies!

RELATIONSHIPS WITH STATUTORY BODIES

Overall, our contacts and relationships with the statutory bodies, such as the Commission for Social Care Inspection and its predecessors, were satisfactory. However, on some inspection visits we found a few inspectors lacking in knowledge about mental health and they were prescriptive in their approach. On those occasions, we took the opportunity to increase their knowledge base by facilitating sensitive discussions and presenting cogent arguments of why we needed to work with flexibility as long as our service principles were sound.

For those inspectors who were patronising and condescending in attitude, we adopted a highly professional and collaborative approach and ensured that they learned some new values in the process.

CONCLUSION

We established the service with trepidation, but never moved away from our primary aspiration to provide a quality service for one of society's most vulnerable groups. The following comments, randomly taken from the visitors' book, demonstrate to a large degree that we were successful in translating our aspirations into an operational framework which delivered a first-class service for people with mental illness.

> 'Wonderful feeling, beautiful location, one of the finest examples of care ethics and property I have ever witnessed.'

> 'If only there were more places like this – so welcoming. A risk well taken.'

> 'Such a beautiful place, such dignity . . . R . . . was so impressed by the atmosphere. Thankfully Tony . . . you had your dream realized.'

> 'A "gift" to see my brother in his new home and a reminder that there is always gold in the shadows.'

> 'It is so refreshing to know that there are still people in the mental health service with ideals and values.'

These few excerpts from the visitors' book, written by professional visitors, relatives and residents, reflect the positive culture, climate and therapeutic environment which we hoped would be realised when we first set out to establish the service. The truth is that, on objective evaluation – both statutory and informal – we exceeded our aspirations and feel proud to have been associated with the initiative. Abbeyfield Lodge changed hands in the latter part of 2005 and we wish the new owners well and feel confident that they will enhance the already well-established services.

What can we share with aspiring entrepreneurs who wish to establish such a service? What worked for us is respect for basics and being in tune with the psychological and physical needs of people. Any good service should be able to demonstrate the following:
➤ ability of staff to anticipate needs
➤ ability to communicate the right information at the right time
➤ supporting feedback systems

➤ absolute integrity when dealing with financial affairs of vulnerable people
➤ briefing relatives about changes and progress
➤ respecting and trusting your staff
➤ effective monitoring of service delivery
➤ an ethos of compassion, inclusion and fairness
➤ promoting loyalty to the service
➤ a real commitment to wanting to change the situation of people who feel institutionally dependent to one which allows individuals to reclaim their identity
➤ a real effort to build links with the local community.

From an idea to a workable plan . . . to an operational framework, we translated an aspiration into a first-class service for people with mental illness.

CHAPTER 13

A space for creativity and healing: Artists in Mind and the mental health system

JOHN HOLT

John Holt writes a passionate piece which expresses his aim in using art and creativity as part of the healing process, but the practical elements are also well-represented – and in some exacting settings.

A NATURAL WORLD VIEW

'We believe that the arts and humanities are a more natural home for such expressions of life's diversity and that the creative ways in which individuals make meaning in their lives and construct their own systems of beliefs, values and goals for themselves, is honored and best understood in a context that does not reduce expressions of humanity to judgments of pathology, deviance and aberrations from the "normal". This is in marked contrast to the language of health care and medicine which necessarily measures the individual according to normative, standardized schemas of development and pre-conceived definitions of health and pathology. We believe that essential freedoms are lost when individual ways of thinking, perceiving and behaving are "managed", and when differences between people are conceptualized in terms of "illness", "pathology" or "disorder"'.

From the ASPA (Academy for the Study of the Psychoanalytic Arts)
www.academyanalyticarts.org/index.htm Reproduced with permission.

The above is the mission statement of the Academy for the Study of the Psychoanalytic Arts which, when I read it some years ago, resonated with what I felt was the central ethos of Artists in Mind (AIM), an arts and mental health charity that I had started some five years previously. Another quote which in many ways exemplified the ethos of AIM was taken with permission from a book by Sean McNiff (Sean McNiff PhD, ATR, is the Provost and Dean of Endicott College in Beverly, Massachusetts). His quotation heads our stationery and declares our intentions within the field of mental well-being.

> 'Whenever illness is associated with loss of soul, the arts emerge spontaneously as remedies, soul medicine. Pairing art and medicine stimulates the creation of a discipline through which imagination treats itself and recycles its vitality back into daily life.'
>
> **McNiff S. *Art as Medicine: creating a therapy of the imagination.* Boston, MA: Shambhala Publications Inc.; 1992. Reproduced with permission.**

Until recently I was a lecturer in Fine Art at Bretton Hall College of the University of Leeds and then at Leeds University School of Fine Art, History of Art and Cultural Studies. I have always held the belief that art, an outcome of the creative process, should be about transformation. By that I mean the often subtle capacity for personal change through creativity. I believe that the formation of language is inherent, but often repressed by childhood experiences. The function of the creative process is to identify, construct and interpret the maps of our life journeys, to utilise language and symbol as a means of orientation, as a mythological apparatus for the guidance of the individual and for the community. Language articulates experience and where language is absent there is a block in the processing of psychic experience.

I have a developing concept that 'creativity is the immune system of the mind and the source of the mythic' and that creativity has a natural tendency, an inclination, when stimulated and encouraged, towards a heightened sense of 'self-realisation' in the individual. This is, I believe, a process of clarification of the relationship between self and the world (e.g. self and body, self and environment, self and God), and it manifests in diverse ways through the construction of language and symbols. In some ways this relates to aspects of the Gestalt school of thought. (Gestalt therapies hold that a person's inability to successfully integrate the parts of their personality into a healthy whole may lie at the root of psychological disturbance. In therapy, the analyst encourages the client to release their emotions, and to recognise these emotions for what they are. Gestalt psychology has been thought of as analogous to field physics.)

I have also been concerned with the élitist status of both the arts and academic life. My research and writing was in areas of the 'other', the 'marginalised', the 'outsider' and, it would seem, the 'un-forgiven'. I worked with Native American, Australian Aboriginal and South Asian arts and artists, and continue to do so. Writing articles and organising tours of artists and works by non-Western artists and scholars, I was drawn to the spiritual and political in both the sacred traditions and the struggle for cultural survival, aspects which so often merged in a desperate longing for 'self-determination', always wary, however, of the dangers of exoticisation and the misrepresentation of others. It was the case that the results of the demeaning of people's identities developed in racism, and indeed genocide and the humiliation of cultures and individuals, clearly resulted in profound psychic damage and this led me to see this as a problem of injury to the human spirit, and hence of the human soul. This area is Jung's territory and his assertion of the struggle for soul led him to ponder the implications of this situation.

'Today this eruption of destructive forces has already taken place, and man suffers from it in spirit. That is why patients force the psychotherapist into the role of a priest, and expect and demand of him that he shall free them from their distress. That is why we psychotherapists must occupy ourselves with problems which, strictly speaking, belong to the theologian.'

From: Jung CJ. *Modern Man in Search of a Soul.*
Harcourt Brace and Company; 1993.

ARTISTS IN MIND: A CREATIVE SANCTUARY

After taking early retirement from Leeds University, I founded the charity called Artists in Mind (AIM), to sustain and develop the work that I had begun in Rampton Secure Hospital (see below). This work took many directions, including the intention to publish works by artists who had experiences of trauma and crisis and for whom art-making had had a significant place in their coping. We work in hospitals, initiating spaces for creativity and healing in projects with artists and service users, all of course limited not by intent but by funding. At AIM, we do not encourage the label 'mental illness' and prefer to speak of individuals as being 'in emotional and spiritual crisis', which in some ways alludes to a causation and an often temporary period of distress and anguish that people experience in a variety of ways. The mental health system is seen as a dark and often unconsidered aspect of our society onto which the public – often fuelled by the media – project their fears of the 'dangerous and the uncontrollable'. This attitude only compounds the sense of alienation and disconnection of the patient and the 'user of mental health services', further driving them into the status of an underclass whose members are required to live in deprived areas where drug dealers and other exploiters of human vulnerability prowl and prey. Even in cases where good work is done by organisations such as AIM, this throwing of the defenceless into exploitative environments only re-traumatises hyper-sensitive individuals.

We at AIM are neither psychotherapists nor theologians, nor do we claim to be; indeed we are at pains to say that we are just artists working with other artists, some of whom are identified as having what the medical model would define as a 'mental illness'. This distinction is important in relation to the reality of the members of AIM (although some of our mentors and artists do have a background in mental health, they work within AIM as artists). And it is significant in relation the mental health system, in that we do not identify 'pathologies' but in fact validate aspects of what mental health professionals might see as indicators of illness. We do this by creating the conditions in which service users' often deep psychological experiences are manifest into symbolic form, as art. The inherent capacity and need to create a symbolic language is, in our opinion, an intrinsic aspect within everyone and particularly when there is psychic disorientation or a loss of self. The outcome of an enhancement, a growth of language, is a development towards 'self-realisation'. As I stated in my book:

> 'Self-realisation or self-integration can be said to be a tendency, a movement towards a greater understanding and acknowledgement of self in relation to the world. Self-realisation in this context does not imply total understanding, but more an improvement in the awareness of self and a reconstruction of awareness of one's relationship with the environmental, personal milieu and history of the individual which charts the route of one's life journey. This was done using the templates of mythology as a guide. The journey is, in this very process, enhanced by self-initiated and archetypal use of images and symbols which acts as a form of mapping in relation to mnemonic and re-collective experiences, and which also includes a future potential.'
>
> **Holt J. *Ways of Knowing: science and mysticism today.***
> **Imprint Academic; 2005. Reproduced with permission.**

WORKING WITHIN SECURE SETTINGS

As a feature of my concerns with the application of the arts to self and community in what I have already defined as an art which transforms, I began to take students into Rampton Secure Hospital. Rampton together with Ashworth and Broadmoor had previous connotations as places for the 'criminally insane'. Here truly were housed the 'un-forgiven'. These are institutions whose captive populations were – and still are – much misrepresented and demonised, particularly by the media. I led workshops there in 'free drawing' and invited writers, artists and international curators into the hospital to work and discuss with the artists/patients the value of the arts and its implications for the psyche. Exhibitions of the artists'/patients' creative output were toured and well received by a public moved, it seemed, by the honesty and integrity of the work. More than this, I made friendships with patients whom I perceived as artists, creative individuals, most of whom had experienced terrible trauma and abuse in their lives and who were damaged – in a post-crisis state – as a result. Many of these artists/patients had 'turned to creativity' only when confined to the forensic hospital, their art-making becoming their own self-regulatory therapy which gave them a dimension of understanding that they had never experienced before. Art became a tool of their healing, supported by such compassionate and inspirational art teachers as Alison Wickstead, whose work at Rampton Hospital created the conditions for transformation, albeit with little managerial acknowledgement of its significance. The people who understand and value such work are the patients themselves, to whom she has given the opportunities to develop a creative language to serve the healing of their emotional and mental health.

> 'Since creativity is the prime mode of communication, it might well be an antidote to violence.'
>
> **Shoham SG. *Art, Crime and Madness.* Eastbourne:**
> **Sussex Academic Press; 2003. Reproduced with permission.**

Violence as a consequence of trauma (in its widest sense) is directed not always outwards but sometimes inwards to self; this is evident not only in the case of patients but also, as already stated, in the case of people bereft of their spiritual traditions and life ways – as with the native peoples of the world. It seemed to me that secure forensic hospitals, with their culture of constant pathologisation and an over-dependency upon pharmaceutical solutions to personal trauma, often only make things worse. (I do believe that there is a sea change underway in the forensic psychiatric system towards a more holistic and expanded acceptance of the nature of the person, but there is still

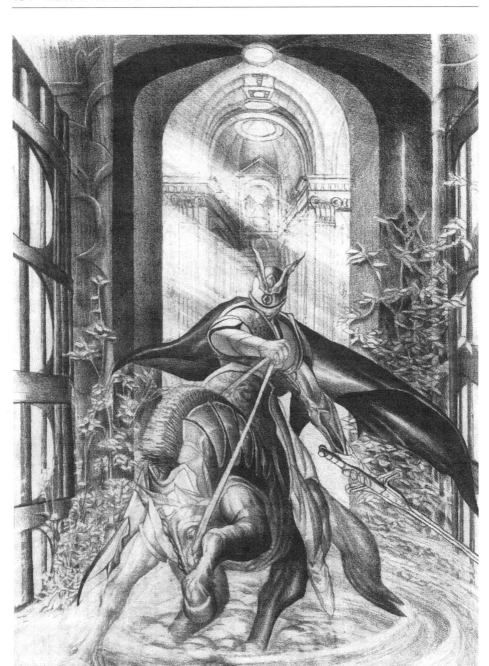

FIGURE 13.1 *Return from Darkness* by Minder Singh © 2004. Pencil drawing with digital enhancement, 30cm × 42cm.

a long way to go.) Drugs can help in terms of the stabilisation of distressing conditions, but should only be used for such purpose. There should, I feel, be an attitude of finding the optimum point where medication provides stability, then other, more conscious talking and creative therapies can be adopted to address the life story, narratives and deep traumas of the individual. I recognise that society needs to be protected against people who are in a phase of cumulative trauma and crisis, just as these unfortunate people need to protected against society. However, the model I advocate is one of a refuge, a sanctuary of compassion and creativity in which they may recover. I have concerns about certain aspects of the ethos and culture of the secure hospitals. Although I have met there individuals of great compassion and commitment to the healing of the patients, they remain, it seems, somewhat at odds with the predominant model of psychiatrist-led objectification of the individual as a merely bio-chemical entity. And while I have seen examples of real progress being made in the quality of lives of patients, I think that enlightened staff who have the time and inclination to listen and to support are often the key to individual healing.

We are not art therapists at AIM; it seems to us that art therapy raises more questions than it answers. We are not therapists but initiators of the therapeutic process, merely by trusting the construction of language in an environment of faith and respect, without analysis or judgement, but, of course with conversations, dialogue and friendship.

THE LIVING MUSEUM: A MODEL OF EXCELLENCE

In 2002 I had the privilege to visit the Living Museum, an extraordinary initiative within a psychiatric institution in Queens, New York, to write a review of an exhibition called *In the Flow: Artists from the Living Museum*, for an international arts journal, *Raw Vision*. The Living Museum is within the grounds of Creedmoor, a vast, downsized psychiatric hospital. The Museum offers a unique programme that exemplifies the convictions that people with what is defined as 'mental illness' are neither simply the embodiment of nor limited by their illness, and that the positive aspect of crisis can be enhanced creativity (if only individuals are given the chance to produce it). The Living Museum is housed in what was the old kitchen and dining area for its then 1350 patients. Two artists, Bolek Greczynski and Dr Janos Marton – a Pole and a Hungarian respectively, the latter also a psychologist – founded the Living Museum. Sadly Bolek died in 1994, but Janos continues the work to this day.

'. . . I began to understand that people with mental illness are blessed with special gifts in the arts. When this gift is organised, channelled, and focussed, it creates art that is significant. "Use your vulnerability as a weapon," Bolek suggested; this remains the museum's guiding motto. Every individual's disadvantage in the museum is re-evaluated and turned to an advantage. To sign an artwork, to step into the limelight, is also a step along the continuum of emancipation and healing. The leap into the public sphere is not easy for everyone. In some cases, the work has to remain anonymous, representing not the individual, but the individual creative spirit.'

Marton J. *In the Flow: artists from the Living Museum.* Catalogue; 2002.
Reproduced with permission.

The Living Museum is an asylum in the true sense; it is a refuge from oppression, a place of sanctuary and, in this case, a space for 'art and healing'. It remains a model of inspiration for me and for my work within AIM. Dr Janos Marton does not claim miraculous transformations through art; the major transformation, he said, comes about by the shift in definition of self from psychiatric patient to artist, thereby changing one's relationship with society, with the world.

There is, I think, much more to explore and recover about the nature of the visionary aspects of the mind than its contemporary psychiatric reduction to a diagnosis of psychosis within the prevailing model of psychiatry. Vision comes to some in a momentary instant, and in many cultures is sought as a means of 'knowing'. In our own culture we label and perceive no value in 'seers', relegating them to a pathological status and labelling them as schizophrenics or psychotics. Of course, not all experiences of this kind can be labelled as mystical – some are experiences of terror and lead to acts of violence against self and others – but we seem to throw the baby out with the bathwater in reducing all psychic experiences as evidence of illness.

Cultures throughout the world describe illness as a loss of soul, a dislocation from the spirits. Although the soul cannot be lost in a literal sense, the need to bring back into balance mind and body, and mind and environment, is the very basis of healing. Only then can the soul be nourished and, indeed, acknowledged. There are many perceptive, sensitive and injured people who, as a consequence of their sensitivities, have insights devoid of the egocentricities of the majority. These sensitive individuals, it seems, pay the price for their vulnerability and, as Bolek – one of the founders of the Living Museum – said, they should 'use their vulnerabilities as a weapon' to sensitise the community through art, through the construction of a language of the inner self. This is 'art of the insane', as Dr Prinzhorn – the founder of the Prinzhorn Collection, set

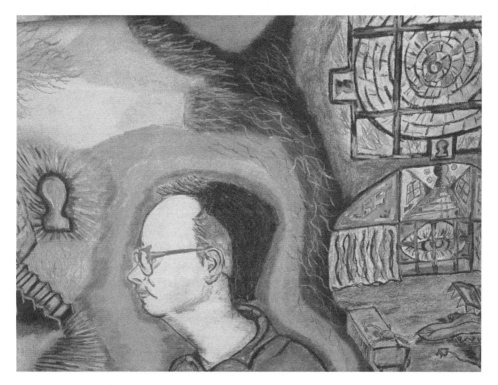

FIGURE 13.2 *Looking to a Bright Future* by Sebastian Wilbur. Reproduced with kind permission.

up in the early 20th century – expressed it. During its search for authentic art at the beginning of the 20th century, the Modern movement discovered not only 'primitive art' and children's drawings, but also 'psychotic art'. Simultaneous to this, a number of psychiatrists began eagerly to collect their patients' pictorial works, although this was principally in the hope that these could be used to assist diagnosis. I believe that such art is an art of authenticity and significance for us all. Art has always had some connotation with madness; well, let the mad reclaim the fertile ground for the benefit of us all!

And so we have it. The dispossessed, the demonised, the 'mentally ill', the un-forgiven. Let us all not turn away from those who, for so many reasons, plunge into crisis; they just might have something valid to tell us all – if only we would listen!

HEALING THROUGH CREATIVITY

In the book *Ways of Knowing: science and mysticism today*, I wrote a chapter entitled 'Creativity as the immune system of the mind and the source of the mythic', in which I addressed the question of how the formation of language can transform and enhance 'self-realisation' in the individual. I was in this inspired by a quote from Arthur Koestler who, in 1975, wrote: 'There is no sharp dividing line between self-repair and self-realisation. All creative activity is a kind of do-it-yourself therapy, an attempt to come to terms with trauma-tising challenges.'[1]

My concern was to ask how the practice evident in AIM's work related to the human condition and particularly for those defined as 'mentally ill'. I developed my argument:

> 'There has always been a human concern with the "fractured self", right from the beginning of human consciousness. Questions fermented in the psyche: what constituted the fissure within and between minds and bodies, what is its causation and how do we repair the damage? And further, how do we reconcile the boundaries within us all, our environment and within the cosmos, between other beings and the spirits, and when things go wrong how do we rectify the imbalance, the illness? These dilemmas were addressed, until the development of the modern world, as spiritual problems with a divine process for healing. To be disconnected and dislocated from the notion of self in the deepest sense of the word is to be deprived of our potential as human beings and to be deluded into perceiving the world as a distorted and hostile place.
>
> Self-realisation or self-integration can be said to be a tendency, a movement towards a greater understanding and acknowledgement of self in relation to the world. Self-realisation in this context does not imply total understanding, but more an improvement in the awareness of self and a reconstruction of awareness of one's relationship with the environmental, personal milieu and history of the individual which charts the route of one's life journey. This was done using the templates of mythology as a guide. The journey is, in this very process, enhanced by self-initiated and archetypal use of images and symbols which acts as a form of mapping in relation to mnemonic and re-collective experiences, and which also includes a future potential.'
>
> **Holt J. *Ways of Knowing: science and mysticism today.***
> **Imprint Academic; 2005. Reproduced with permission.**

There is always suspicion – and indeed a perceived threat – to therapeutic practice that challenges the bastions of the mental health system. There is clearly a dominance of security over therapy in many forensic settings, manifest in the disproportional spending and dominance of decisions in favour of security over the therapeutic, and in the managerial decision-making dominance of security, which can sometimes eclipse innovative and significant healing initiatives. This has come about from subsequent governmental 'knee-jerk reactions' to past incidents in relation to forensic psychiatric care. It is often in the initial, primary phase of psychic imbalance where people are failed as they experience an acute phase in their equilibrium and are not fully supported through it. There is an immediate need for high support in the acute phases of disorientation and this is not always evident.

There are other similar arts organisations to AIM – foundations such as the Lankelly-Chase Foundation, which has targeted the much-neglected arts provision in secure forensic settings, particularly for women, as an area of specific concern, and charities who give support and funding to arts organisations who work in this sector. This has been clearly indicated in the support given by the management at Rampton Hospital and within Nottinghamshire NHS Trust for two long-term projects with two nationally and internationally significant sculptural artists, Halima Cassell and Brendan Hesmondhalgh. The two landmark projects involved two 20-week residencies with the two experienced professional artists, resulting in the acquisition by both male and female patients of skills in visual research, drawing and sculpture. The patients developed the work together with their nursing and support staff and the end product was taken away from the hospital and cast to a very high professional standard. The outcome is to be two major site-specific sculptural works, which will enhance the hospital environment for staff, visitors and most importantly patients, enriching the hospital in a permanently uplifting way. This project was made possible with funding from the Arts Council and Nottinghamshire NHS Trust and support from the staff and managers of the hospital. AIM hopes that the success of this project will lead to further partnerships working with both Rampton and other high-security and medium-security hospitals. Working in this way in secure hospitals is a complex and at times taxing endeavour. The tight restrictions on materials and equipment, particularly in relation to the women patients, did interfere somewhat with their capacity to produce work and we did lose sessions for what seemed like matters of hospital management and supervision and not concerns with the delivery of the arts experiences, but the patients and staff who participated all benefited clearly from the experience. In sculpture sessions, AIM would not allow any staff to stand around passively observing the creative process but we insisted that everyone participate in the sessions as artists; indeed the situation arose where patients helped staff who were not as fluent in their creativity. These landmark projects have opened the door to the value and significance of high-quality arts experiences in secure hospitals. The two major works resulting from these projects will clearly enhance the aesthetic and spiritual environment of the hospital.

THE HEALING SPACE

As McNiff observes, the 'classifying mind' has used pathology to further its schemes and it is the presumption that the well heal the sick, but the system itself can said to be pathological. As McNiff states, 'When staff openly accept the pathology of their interactions with one another, then the system is ready for transformation'.[1] This resonates with work being done into the nature of the 'wounded healer', in which those who have experienced deep trauma themselves made empathetic and compassionate healers. Although this may well be regarded as a subjective realm in relation to the mental health system, it can be argued that this system is in itself subjective and that mental diagnoses are imprecise and subject to continual challenge and conjecture. In this context, what is most effective is for the patient to have a deep trust and respect for the healer who is working with them. By paying attention to our experiences, learning the ways of releasing them, and understanding the art of spiritual transformation, we can lift up all woundedness and enter the realms of light. The 'artists as healers' can be said to be more capable of understanding the seeming irrational narratives of so-called 'mentally ill' individuals. In both hospital and the community, the success of schemes which give deference to and respect for those so defined falls into this area of the creation of a sanctuary or healing space. When AIM works in secure hospitals, the patients, nurses, escorts and management are all told that, within the space of art-making, they are all artists. The normal roles of patient, nurse, doctor and so on dissipate in an albeit temporary shift to a state of 'artistic egalitarianism' devoid of the status that the institution has constructed. This democratic sanctuary refreshes and enlivens all participants – indeed it is often the case that a patient ends up supporting and encouraging the staff in their art-making. This does not undermine the necessary structures of the hospital but gives temporary respite from its conventions, to the psychological benefit of all.

One particular model in relation to an artistic sanctuary initiated by AIM carried out the placement of the acute and long-term ill into artists' studios. There provision existed for mentoring, materials and professional development of the service users who re-defined themselves as artists and adjusted their lives accordingly. This particular scheme, entitled the Service User Mentor Scheme (SUMS), began over two years ago with a little funding from the Arts Council and Awards for All and developed from previous work

I had done in Wakefield with a group of post-institutionalised service users who felt bereft of support in their creativity and art-making once they had left the psychiatric hospital.

CONCLUSION

In conclusion one might simply ask the following questions: How does art heal? and What are the implications of art and creativity for mental health services in the UK today? Some scientific studies tell us that art heals by changing a person's physiology and attitude. Work done in the US talks about the reopening of pathways in the brain which had been sealed off by trauma before the trialling of creative activities. When one is in a mindset of creativity, it is true that the body's physiology changes from one of stress and fracture to one of deep relaxation, from one of fear to one of creativity and inspiration. Creativity transfers an individual into a different brainwave pattern; art and music affect a person's autonomic nervous system, their hormonal balance and their brain neurotransmitters. Research has also has shown that art and music affect every cell in the body instantly to create a healing physiology that changes the immune system and blood flow to all organs of the body. Art-making can also change a person's perceptions of their world, developing increased self-realisation. Further, the practice of art and music changes the community status of an individual defined as 'mentally ill' into that of a person who contributes to the *Zeitgeist* (the spirit of the age) of contemporary society in which they live. This contribution can often take the mental patient or the service user labelled with paranoid schizophrenia or personality disorder to the status of an artist who illuminates, moves or challenges an audience, sharing deep, beautiful or fearful insights into the human condition. As artists, these individuals then undergo change in their attitude and emotional state, developing self-esteem, confidence and a real sense of self-worth. This creates hope and positivity, with the newly designated artists in turn being able to help other people to cope with difficulties, as wounded yet knowledgeable healers in their own right. Art practice can thus transform a person's outlook and way of being in the world and make a powerful contribution to the spiritual health of the community.

REFERENCES

1 Reprinted by permission of PFD on behalf of the Estate of Arthur Koestler © 1967. *The Ghost in the Machine.* Pan Books Ltd.
2 McNiff S. *Art as Medicine: creating a therapy of the imagination.* Boston, MA: Shambhala Publications Inc.; 1992, p. 25.

CHAPTER 14

Enhancing the healing environment

SHARON SQUIRES and DEBORAH THOMPSON

The importance of the environment in the context of treatment has become increasingly recognised. This chapter, written by two senior nurses, shows that the very process of re-examining a ward, and its functions and spaces, can change attitudes and significantly improve care.

BACKGROUND

In September 2003 the Commission for Health Improvement (CHI) published a report into allegations of physical and emotional abuse of vulnerable older people by staff on Rowan Ward in Manchester, a mental health unit for older people run by Manchester Mental Health and Social Care Trust.[1] What resulted from this report was a coordinated review of Hospital Trusts to identify any clinical areas that may be at risk from developing problems similar to Rowan Ward, and to form an action plan and to address such problems.

Inpatient areas within Nottinghamshire Healthcare NHS Trust, like those of many Trusts across the country, were visited by the Strategic Health Authority (SHA) during March 2005. The purpose of these visits was to meet with ward managers and collate information relating to the themes identified in the Rowan report.

The issues identified during the SHA's visits highlighted some good practice and some pockets of excellence within the service. Conversely, the SHA also perceived a service without purpose, lacking an overall vision, introspective and seen as dragging its feet and not keeping up with the sweeping demands of the new National Health Service (NHS). This negative image was believed to be influencing staff in their approach to care and their ability to work effectively with other agencies. In identifying these challenges and the need for service changes, we recognised that we had an opportunity to influence the way our practice was being instigated as well as casting off the negative images associated with mental health services for older people. Moreover, older persons' services were undergoing something of a transformation due to the closure of beds and relocation of services to provide a more specialised model of inpatient care.

A positive outcome of this review was the suggestion by the SHA that we apply to the King's Fund for inclusion on their Enhancing the Healing Environment programme – a suggestion which we readily pursued.

And so began our journey to influence our culture and practice so that we could provide services in an environment of which we would all be proud. For us, it was not just an opportunity to address issues of the environment in which we cared for older people, but a timely vehicle by which to drive forward a person-centred approach to care.

ENHANCING THE HEALING ENVIRONMENT AND THE KING'S FUND

'We know that the environment where you are treated makes a difference to how you feel and in some cases how quickly you recover.

For too long mental health facilities were neglected and this programme is just one sign that things are changing for the better. We believe this will make a real difference both to patients and to the staff who take part.'

Niall Dickson, Chief Executive, King's Fund

Dickson N. Patients and staff to benefit from £1.2 million programme to improve mental health hospitals.

Press release. London: King's Fund; 15 December 2005.

The King's Fund was founded in 1897 as an independent charitable foundation working to improve health services to poor people in London. Since the advent of the NHS, the King's Fund began to focus its expertise and resources on developing good practice in the NHS, for example through training courses, and on grants designed to support new initiatives. One such initiative is the Enhancing the Healing Environment (EHE) programme.

EHE encourages and enables nurse-led teams to work in partnership with patients and carers to improve the environment in which they deliver care. The programme consists of two main elements:

➤ a development programme for the multi-disciplinary project team, nurse led and including estates and facilities staff, arts coordinators, patients and strategic health authority representatives
➤ a £35 000 grant to undertake a project to enhance the healing environment (£30 000 from the King's Fund and £5000 from each participating Trust).

NOTTINGHAMSHIRE HEALTHCARE NHS TRUST – THE PROJECT TEAM

Each EHE project is initially required to conduct a feasibility survey to identify an appropriate area within their service to 'enhance', and subsequently to submit frequent and detailed reports to the King's Fund in order to gain their approval at each stage of the project and, ultimately, to secure the release of the grant monies. To pursue this, we assembled a multi-disciplinary project team.

OUR JOURNEY THROUGH THE EHE PROGRAMME

After attending the launch of the EHE programme in London, and having met as a group to discuss our passion for making a difference, we recognised our potential to become an effective team. Our strengths lay in our commitment, energy, resourcefulness and ingenuity. Although the team was required to identify and develop only one area within our service, our involvement on this project fuelled our aspirations to influence the wider healthcare environment.

Each team member brought differing but equally valuable skill sets to the project, enabling us to take on specific roles and responsibilities whilst our project leader (Sharon Squires) kept her eyes on the horizon and our feet on the ground. We readily acknowledge that the success of the project is entirely dependent on user satisfaction, and that considerable energy needed to be invested in forging links with service users, carers and staff, from the outset. A successful outcome also depended on meeting the criteria laid down by the King's Fund and working within the constraints of the £35 000 budget.

WHERE? AND WHY?

The team considered a number of locations where we could effectively 'enhance the healing environment'. Initially we considered creating a social space in an area which linked a new Private Finance Initiative (PFI) built ward to an existing ward. However, the future usage of this area became uncertain, so we had to think again. Next, we considered improving another of our Mental Health Services for Older People wards at the St Francis Unit within Nottingham City Hospital. Once more, we found a lack of clarity over the future use of these wards.

Finally the team elected to undertake the EHE project on Silver Birch Ward, a recently completed PFI build. The new Silver Birch Ward, to which users and staff had just transferred, replaced a very old ward, built as part of the original workhouse at the Highbury site. Silver Birch already had a pleasing environment, due in part to its 'newness' and also because of the clever use of colour and fittings. The ward area is very large and split into four main zones, with each zone colour coordinated to represent a season. For example, blue was used as the main colour theme at the ward entrance, representing winter. By using colour to identify care zones, there was already a clear theme to the ward which assisted with way-finding and gave each care zone individuality. Following initial discussions with carers, staff and relatives, we were convinced that our £35 000 King's Fund project could enhance what was already there and give us the greatest opportunity to provide the 'wow' factor within our modest budget.

However, it is important to mention at this juncture that whilst our plans were ambitious and exciting, we had to be mindful of the sensitivities which surrounded us at that time. The unit was experiencing major organisational change; patients who had lived on the ward for many years were being discharged under the continuing care criteria into appropriate care homes. This inevitably caused anxieties for their carers and relatives, who were naturally preoccupied with issues relating to possible changes in care settings that lay ahead for them and their loved ones. Staff on the ward were not only dealing with this sensitive issue but also making the physical move from one care environment to another. So, to introduce our exciting new plans for EHE into the mix at this stage was, of course, extremely challenging for all involved.

SILVER BIRCH WARD

Silver Birch Ward has 22 en-suite bedrooms and caters for older people with mental health needs. The colourful design scheme already featured artworks created by users of our adult mental health services, and a number of mosaics were created in a participatory workshop attended by patients, relatives and ward staff. This workshop acted as an initiation for the project. Although not directly linked to our project, it acted as a driver for the future involvement of users, carers and staff and helped us to initiate a collaborative transition from old to new.

Since the completion of Silver Birch Ward, the project team spent some time absorbing this new environment and concluded that we could usefully impact (and provide the 'wow') in a number of areas – namely the approach to the entrance, the main door, reception area, the visitors' room, the dining room and adjacent patio. Our goal was to add value to what is essentially the blank canvas of a generic PFI build. The build quality was of a very high standard, but nevertheless attracted comments from visitors and carers as being 'clinical'. We hoped, therefore, to improve the character of the space so that it met the needs of patients, carers and staff – reflecting what they would expect to enjoy in a 'first-class lounge' environment, for example.

Based on feedback from users and carers, we considered the specifics of exactly what we were aiming to do in these chosen areas. We needed to soften the impact of the entrance by looking at ways of making it more welcoming, thereby creating a better first impression. We needed to give clear signage to facilitate a natural flow from one part of the environment to another, guiding visitors in the right direction (described recently by one carer as a 'fear of not knowing what lies beyond'). We aimed to achieve this by providing visual contrast, using colour and lighting to promote recognition of objects and drawing the eye towards and away from areas.

We also needed to give a clear signal to people to utilise areas such as the visitors' room, and to create a welcoming environment which communicated and provided a positive reaction. We learnt that it was not sufficient simply to hang artistic designs on the walls, but to consider carefully the positioning, adequate lighting and an acknowledgement of who had created the work – all of which serve to encourage people to pause and look at the art. Lighting is a particularly important aspect for our patients and visitors, as research indicates that older people need three times the amount of light to see as clearly as younger people. Consideration also needed to be given to the balance of peace and privacy with high-activity stimulating areas and the need to tailor the environment to the needs of our dementia clients, enabling maximum independence and a sense of personhood.

In order to achieve some of the above we had to consider the functionality of each space, negotiate its use and think carefully how each area would link together with the others.

In an attempt to formulate ideas to put out for consultation, we explored the use of thematic designs depicting 'Silver Birch'. Like a silver thread, perhaps. Such a simple device could tie in the design elements throughout the ward, providing the direction-finding function previously mentioned. We envisioned a silver thread starting at the ward entrance and weaving its way through the common areas.

GIVERS AND RECIPIENTS OF CARE

Dementia care wards have long been associated with draconian services which have not had the benefit of major investment over the years. Moreover, staff working in these areas are afforded little credibility within the hierarchy of nursing. Even now when newly qualified nurses are complaining of the lack of vacancies within the NHS, we continue to find that very few newly qualified staff choose to specialise in dementia care. Certainly dementia nursing would appear less glamorous than, say, acute care or forensic nursing. The skills required by those staff caring for people with dementia are not easily categorised or measured. This kind of nursing requires absolute devotion from the caregiver and the ability to care for someone unconditionally. Often the work is dirty and physically demanding.

People admitted onto the ward have a variety of needs, which are often challenging and complex and which require a variety of skills from the care team. Sometimes their behaviour is unpredictable; they may be aggressive, confused and distressed. Our aim is to work with the individual to promote their level of well-being, foster their selfhood and help them to maintain optimum levels of ability. The people who are admitted onto the ward usually are at the middle to late stages of dementia. Our role on Silver Birch Ward is to maintain quality of life in a safe environment. Dementia not only affects the person but it also has an impact on their family and friends. We acknowledge the importance of enabling families to remain active participants in the dementia sufferer's life and want to foster an inclusive, family-orientated approach to care.

THE IMPORTANCE OF ENVIRONMENT

Our intention through enhancing the healing environment is to create an enriched living and working space that brings together elements of good design, art and quality. What this project allows us to do is to develop the environment in a way that challenges an institutional approach to hospital environments. One element of quality of life we considered to be important was the issue of a family-orientated, inclusive approach to care. When people visit they want spaces where they are not excluded from others. Also, and most importantly, we wanted to enable carers and friends who visit to be able to sit, perhaps with other carers, and feel that they were not isolated from the general 'goings on' around them. This was of particular concern to some of our carers, as they felt that the old ward had provided this and the new ward did not. We had also checked out our ideas and found that there was a lot more to creating a good environment for people with dementia. International literature on principles for designing specific facilities was summarised by Marshall,[2] concluding that accommodation for people with dementia should:

➤ compensate for disability
➤ maximise independence, reinforce personal identity and self-esteem/ confidence
➤ demonstrate care for staff
➤ be orientating and understandable
➤ welcome relatives and the local community
➤ control and balance stimuli.

COLLABORATION AND INVOLVEMENT

As mentioned previously, the project came at a time when there were changes to the organisation directly impacting on the staff, users and carers of the ward involved. It had always been our intention to make this project more than just something that influenced the physical environment. We set out with the view to involve staff, users and carers throughout the project.

The team conducted a range of communication activities to 'spread the word' about the anticipated benefits of our project. Each team member had access to a variety of contacts both internally and externally to do this effectively. The project team felt strongly that this project had the potential to be a powerful, cohesive force for very disparate groups working within the Trust, for users and carers of our services and for the community. By engaging supporters and partners we will, we hope, lay the foundations for other projects to grow from our Silver Birch seedling! By adding character and innovative use of space and function, we aim to have a positive influence on the way Silver Birch affects the lives of those who live and work there and for those who visit for a while. Moreover, by speaking loud and proud and by publishing our work we aim to ensure that the culture of EHE gets adopted and embedded in the organisation as a whole.

The project team has worked hard to ensure that it puts the patient at the centre of everything we do, which means:

➤ fostering a culture where listening to patients and carers and acting on their views is an everyday reality which results in real changes
➤ establishing clear and effective mechanisms for involving patients,

carers and communities in decisions about their own health and the environment in which health services are delivered.

We consider ourselves fortunate to have co-opted an excellent and experienced advocate from Age Concern onto the project. Together with a carer representative on the team, this gives a much-needed voice to our patients, who due to the nature of their illness are unable to articulate their own views.

The project team conducted presentations at ward/carers' meetings to discuss our plans and obtain much-valued feedback. The EHE team also attended the Continuing Care Steering Group and fostered links with our PFI partners, with adult mental health service users and local artists. We distributed an environmental questionnaire to all carers, relatives, staff and visitors and collated the results, drawing out key themes to inform our final vision for the project. For example, completed questionnaires described the reception area as being 'impersonal', the ward was seen as 'requiring better signposting', and a sense of disappointment was expressed that the new facility was 'too clinical and has no heart'.

In addition to direct work with carers, the project was presented at a partnership 'away' day where staff were asked to contribute their ideas on what they would do to improve the environment. An interactive project room was set up on Silver Birch Ward to house EHE display materials, and a link was provided on the Trust's intranet site which identified the team and described the aims, objectives and activities of the project.

We were clear from the start of this project that there needed to be a balance between therapeutic risk-taking and patient choice. We did this through representing what the people said they wanted and balancing that against what the Trust said we could have. This is where our skills of communication, negotiation and reasoning were particularly useful. It was imperative that we worked alongside infection control, domestic services and the estates team to get their advice but also to help them to understand the reasons behind our choices and to get them to 'buy into' the project.

The official opening of Silver Birch Ward also gave us further opportunity to present the project to staff, users and carers, builders, architects, facilities staff and our PFI partners. Following an impromptu briefing on our project by the project manager, a very welcome donation of £500 was given that day by a local Freemasons group.

As funds were limited, the team decided that the full services of an architect were not required. However, valuable links were made with eminent academics from the University of Nottingham's Institute of Architecture School of the Built Environment, who have attended several project meetings and provided expert support and advice on our overall project plans and objectives. The project received a further boost with a grant of £20 000 from the Trust Board.

TEAM DEVELOPMENT

The EHE philosophy is about developing not only the environments where we work but also the team and the individuals within that team. Ten months into the project one of the team members left, which provided us with new challenges. Although we acknowledged that a vital link had been lost we were able to take our project forward with enthusiasm. There have been periods when we have disagreed or where one or other of us has had to take a step back because of work pressures. However, as a team we have all been able to contribute something of value to the project. We have learnt that working on a project such as this can conflict with our usual roles and responsibilities, but therein lay the challenge.

CHANGE IN PRACTICE

As part of the project we needed to determine how an enhancement of this space would impact on clinical practice. Independent evaluations of the King's Fund programme have shown that completed projects exhibit a number of emerging themes – the most significant being the 'humanising' of the hospital environment. This has been evidenced by the uplifting effects of artwork, creating distraction and enjoyment, along with the provision of greater privacy and dignity for patients. Significant long-term benefits show increased ownership of the environment and a greater awareness of its impact on the users and employees of the service.

The Department of Health published an evaluation of 23 EHE projects which included the application of the NHS Estates, Achieving Excellence Design Evaluation Toolkit (AEDET) and a Staff and Patient Environment Calibration Tool (ASPECT).[3] These evidenced significant improvement on all measurable indicators once projects were completed, including higher user satisfaction, an increased usage of otherwise underutilised areas, positive changes in working practice and, most importantly, the therapeutic benefits derived from an environment designed by users, carers and staff, which fulfil a fitness for purpose and serve to reduce stress.

For our particular project we aimed to change clinical practice by:

➤ increasing interaction between staff, users and carers, thereby increasing everyone's sense of well-being and ownership of the environment

> developing and redefining spaces, improving the patient journey both physically and emotionally
> improving how people feel about being in care, creating less clinical, calmer spaces
> creating a person-centred environment with emphasis on the experience of positive feeling and improved privacy and dignity.

In order to establish the impact of the changes to the environment on our staff, users and carers, we will carry out a survey after the work is completed. In addition to this we intend to look specifically at how these changes impact on the clinical changes mentioned above. In order to do this we will undertake Dementia Care Mapping,[4] an existing method used in our service to determine the experience of care as perceived by the person with dementia.

For the Trust as a whole, we anticipate that this project will set a benchmark for other building/refurbishment projects. For example, we are utilising new materials and models which could usefully be replicated across the Trust. The project showcases what is possible, raises the profile for arts in healthcare, demonstrates the power of fostering involvement and partnership working, provides positive publicity for the Trust and gives an opportunity for service re-design and environmental improvement to work in tandem – form following function.

DETAILS OF DESIGN
The sum of £35 000 sounds like a great deal of money to enhance an environment. In reality, however, this is a tight budget if you plan to impact on so many areas, as we do.

Our intention is to engender positive feelings about our services before people enter the ward, by utilising the approaching corridor walls to display large photographic prints on canvas to identify 'the work that goes on in the place', i.e. positive images of older people, the staff and carers to set the scene for what goes on inside.

At the main doors we also want to provide an impressive illuminated sign, setting the standard for the rest of the ward and moving away from traditional hospital signage.

As people enter reception they will encounter improved lighting, which enhances the existing artwork with spotlights, and we are creating a welcoming place to sit. In addition, the glass panelling that gives the space a clinical look will be softened with the use of transfers etched onto glass, which will also serve to introduce the Silver Birch thematic design concept. When we talked about the silver thread leading through the ward, this is where it begins. From this point, people's eyes will also be drawn to the first of a series of illuminated glass mosaic art boxes.

As anyone proceeds onto the ward, they will see the second of our illuminated mosaic art boxes, and the silver birch theme carries on down the corridor on the glass panels until the dining room is reached.

The dining room will undergo major transformation. This room has the largest floor space on the ward and leads to an outside terrace. Here we intend to expand the function of the space by clearly defining two areas – one for dining and one for more relaxed eating, coffee or visiting. By providing sofas, we hope to encourage more direct communication and to present a choice from the upright chairs we already have. In addition, we aim to make the adjoining terrace more accessible by installing patio doors – thereby improving the transitional flow from inside to outside.

The dining room will also be enhanced decoratively through the use of colour-coordinated furniture and soft furnishings, to give more of a restaurant feel and less of an institutional feel. The terrace will have an awning to provide shade and shelter, and there will be additional lighting under the fascia to make the space appealing in the evening. From the dining room, a further illuminated mosaic art box will be visible.

CONCLUSION

At the beginning of this chapter, a summary of the services we provided painted something of a gloomy picture. This project has offered an ideal opportunity to develop a positive and forward-looking service. It is too early in the process to measure the real impact of the changes we plan to make; however, as the programme and the project team develop we continue to work within our vision. The challenges we have faced so far have been many. We have learnt not to make assumptions; what we thought was important was often not what the staff and carers viewed as important. When you work in an area, there can be a tendency to miss significant aspects of or become desensitised to the environment. We now know that we can look beyond the traditional and breathe art and life into healthcare environments, creating spaces that not only enhance the patient's journey through our wards but make the latter truly healing environments.

REFERENCES

1 Commission for Health Improvement (CHI) Investigations. *Investigation into matters arising from care on Rowan Ward: Manchester Mental Health and Social Care Trust.* London: HMSO; 2003.

2 Marshall M. Environment: how it helps to see dementia as a disability in care homes and dementia. In: Benson S, editor. *The Journal of Dementia Care Homes and Dementia*; London: Hawker Publications; 2001.

3 Department of Health, King's Fund. *Improving the patient experience – celebrating achievement: enhancing the healing environment programme.* London: HMSO; 2006.

4 Bradford Dementia Group. *Dementia Care Mapping (DCM). DCM 8 Users Manual.* Making Knowledge Work; 2005.

CHAPTER 15

The Retreat: an alternative perspective from the independent sector

JENNY McALEESE

This is an important description of how the current scene appears to a well-established provider of mental health services in the independent sector. Although the national agenda may advocate a significant role for such organsiations, this account suggests the current reality is no more than a reluctant acceptance of their existence.

THE EARLY RETREAT

The Retreat was founded in 1792 by William Tuke, a York Quaker and tea merchant, who set out to treat humanely, respectfully and kindly people suffering from mental illness, paying particular attention to their physical comfort. In an era when almost all such patients were simply locked away in squalor, Tuke created an environment where people could take responsibility for their own emotions and behaviour, gain a clearer sense of themselves and their responsibility towards others and develop trusting relationships which were often a key component of their recovery.

The early Retreat employed few professionally trained staff and functioned very much as a family. 'It was designed to be dwelt in as a large private house. Its atmosphere was domestic, and it was run along paternal lines. The super-intendent and his assistants were the "family", and a spiritual bond was sought between staff and patients.'[1] Its establishment began a revolution in the humane treatment of people suffering from mental illness.

THE RETREAT TODAY

The Retreat today continues to reflect its original principles of humanity, respect, responsibility and minimum restraint, and retains its strong Quaker links and ethos. As in 1792, the success of our work depends on the quality and attitude of the staff team, and The Retreat is fortunate in having a team of dedicated clinicians committed to our work, who believe in the likelihood of change, use support to enable each other to hold on to hope through difficult times and who hold a clear and shared vision linked to our history as well as to contemporary thinking about recovery and what works in the treatment of mental illness.

In the foreword to the *Description of The Retreat*, re-published in 1996, Kathleen Jones writes, 'Respect for patients, the emphasis on human rights and the value placed on relationships are as relevant now as they were in 1813.'[2]

Respecting service users

We believe that one of the best ways of treating service users with respect is to involve them as much as possible, both in their own care and recovery and in the running of services. This is reflected in our recognition of the service user as expert in their illness and in our commitment to being a leader as far as service user involvement is concerned. Whilst The Retreat has a long history of involving service users in their care, it is only fairly recently that we have begun to involve them more in the day-to-day running of the establishment. We have aimed for real service-user involvement, rather than something tokenistic; involvement that enhances the quality of our service, and it is worth noting that what we have achieved has been at little additional cost.

Our next aim is to build on this work and to extend our involvement of family and carers. Trish Cain, our Service User Consultant, writes the following:

MY EXPERIENCE

Although service user involvement (SUI) is still very much in its infancy here at The Retreat, it is quickly gaining momentum with a small but dedicated core committee who are moving SUI forward with the help and support of managers, senior managers and trustees. There is no doubt that it is being embraced by the organisation wholeheartedly.

As I became more involved and attended this year's Mind Conference, which was very much focused on SUI, I realised that The Retreat were fulfilling virtually all the criteria laid down by already successful SUI groups. I was impressed with what was happening at The Retreat and proud to be a part of moving things forward.

Real involvement

The Retreat is encouraging all service users throughout the hospital to become involved at some level . . . from a monthly Service User Forum, which is open to any client to air their views and/or grievances about ANY hospital matter be it big or small . . . up to a place on the Clinical Governance Committee.

Service Users are being asked to take up places on all the sub-groups, to be involved in interviewing all new staff, to be involved in research and also any training taking place.

Already Service Users have attended workshops to help rewrite a Patients' Charter and were invited to attend a workshop to explore how outcomes are measured and what the hospital could learn from hearing what the service users see as *real* outcomes in the way they're able to live their lives . . . and how these two differ.

I was invited to sit on the panel during the formal interviews for a consultant psychiatrist . . . and I can assure you that I was invited and accepted as an equal. I am in no doubt that The Retreat sees SUI as the way forward.

Service users and recovery

There is a widely held belief that each patient is the expert in their own illness and that by using that expertise productively, with help from a wide range of professionals available, the patient is given the best possible chance of recovery. The Retreat is proving to be a great advocate of this way forward.

Having SUI adds other dimensions to the road to recovery . . . empowerment and confidence building being just two of them. I also feel that there is great therapeutic value in being a part of the running of your hospital. Being consulted, being listened to . . . being heard and knowing that it's not just 'lip service' but that your views really do count. This is about patients having a say in what is happening in their care, their hospital and their lives. Having a cross-section of inpatients and ex-patients working together is yet another dimension . . . those still in hospital see at first hand that it is possible to move on and ex-patients find themselves being held as role models for recovery. At the same time those of us who are well into our recovery have a reminder of how far we have come along the road whilst still being involved on a different level with the people and the environment that helped to make it possible.

WHAT MAKES US DIFFERENT

Operating as a not-for-profit independent hospital with a turnover of £8 million and just over 100 beds on two sites in York, The Retreat is very much one of the smaller players in the mental health market-place. Some years ago, like many independent providers, it took the decision to develop specialist niche services, focusing on those areas where service users' needs are not met particularly well by the statutory services. This led us down the route of services for borderline personality disorder, eating disorder, complex psychoses, older patients with challenging behaviour and, in conjunction with another charity, brain injury.

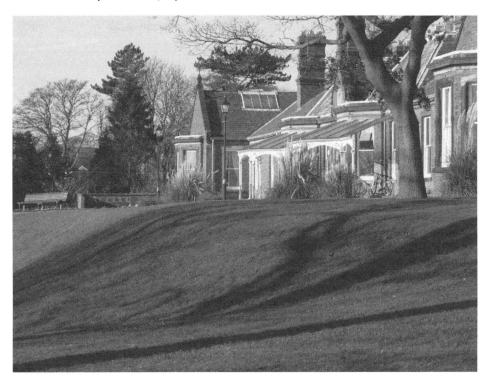

FIGURE 15.1 Naomi Unit at The Retreat, York. Reproduced with kind permission.

What these services have in common is that they tend to admit people who have complex needs and who have had many previous and frequently unsuccessful hospital admissions, usually in National Health Service (NHS) settings. Indeed, The Retreat is often seen as the placement of last resort, which does sometimes put a great deal of pressure on both the service user and the clinical team. The services all have a common approach in that they involve the service user and their family/carer as much as possible, adopt a therapeutic community approach to varying degrees and, perhaps most importantly, do not give up on people. Because of its size and independence, The Retreat is better able than most to devise a service specifically tailored to the needs of the individual and to modify existing or develop new services in response to changing needs.

AN EXAMPLE OF OUR WORK

In our specialist Psychosis and Recovery Unit we focus on the needs of adults with severe psychosis who are usually resistant to conventional psychiatric treatment or at least have not made a complete recovery. We are able to offer a consistent approach with an established team over three to five years, which allows sufficient time to develop a framework of trusting relationships within which we can work psychologically. We have now managed to help a number of people, both young and not so young, to move back into the community successfully.

For example, some years ago we took over the care of a patient with a long-term intractable recurrent psychosis who had been in and out of hospital for years and was referred to us for long-term hospital care. The patient was angry about this view and wanted to go home. That patient has now had four years living independently at home without inpatient care and is about to reapply for a driving licence. After about a year the referring consultant said, 'I don't know what you're doing but I'd like to bottle it' . . . but maybe some of it doesn't go in a bottle.

What we believe we were (and are) doing differently was (and is) attending to key elements of the spiritual dimension, developing trusting relationships, listening, sharing in and bearing some of the pain and loss with both the patient and their elderly mother. This meant, for example, avoiding 'pathologising' all behaviour, not rushing to use the Mental Health Act in an antagonising way, and being open and meeting on equal terms as human beings.

Most of these key elements relate to what can be recognised as central features of spirituality: purpose and meaning; relationships; trust; coming to terms with bereavements; recognising creative needs; finding meaning in madness; journeying through pain; telling stories; an acceptance of the validity of an individual's experience, belief or aspiration; a willingness to help them make some sense of it and an acknowledgement of the spiritual in the real ordinariness of life. Awareness, language and approach are all crucial elements in how this is done.

Links with the National Health Service

The Retreat's links with the NHS go back over thirty years, when it had a contract with Yorkshire Regional Health Authority to care for health professionals and their family members. That work has now more or less disappeared. In the late 1980s and early 1990s, The Retreat took the difficult-to-place service users when the local large psychiatric hospitals were closed and care in the community was introduced. In the late 1990s, when the local services were struggling with a shortage of acute beds and York residents were being sent as far away as Birmingham for inpatient care, The Retreat negotiated an 'overflow' contract with the local Health Authority – a contract that operated until a couple of years ago.

Looking back over these arrangements, they were probably generally far from satisfactory from the point of view of anyone involved, as referral was on the basis of the status of the individual service user (i.e. health professional, inpatient of a hospital that was closing or patient who required inpatient care for whom there was no NHS bed available), rather than after careful consideration of an individual's needs. Today, whilst there remains a small cohort of those service users from the old psychiatric hospitals, contracts with NHS commissioners follow referral of individuals to one of our specialist services, based on a detailed assessment of the individual's needs.

Our experience in relation to the overflow contract was at times disturbing in terms of what it revealed, both about the NHS approach to the independent sector and also sometimes its apparent lack of concern about the best interests of individual service users. The NHS view quite clearly was that we should only be used if there were no NHS beds available and that was absolutely understandable. Less understandable, however, was that as soon as a bed did become available, the NHS would often take back a service user part way through their inpatient stay. This often had negative consequences, particularly when it involved someone in a deep depression in need of peace and quiet being moved to an acute ward full of noisy and aggressive patients experiencing psychosis. Such relapses and extended admissions prevented the NHS from being able to benefit from the investment it had made in purchasing our services.

When we tried to have conversations about appropriate placements, suggesting that we take individuals who were either suffering from depression or making good progress with their recovery from a psychotic episode in order to ensure that incompatible client groups were not mixed, this was interpreted as an unwillingness/inability on our part to take difficult cases. We did, however, persevere and managed to get the appropriate agreements and protocols in place, which meant the individual service user was able to receive continuity of care in the most appropriate setting, and the NHS was able to get value for money from its investment in the independent sector. At the time of writing, it is interesting to note that we are again experiencing a shortage of beds locally, and we are receiving a number of more general acute overflow referrals – this time we have moved quickly to get the protocols in place!

Looking in from the outside, I am often concerned by the apparent lack of an intelligent approach towards cost-saving in the NHS, and I wonder whether the sudden influx of overflow referrals mentioned above is a result of an increase in demand or the stripping out of some services in order to save costs. I am aware of at least one case when a forensic patient was referred to the independent sector because, although there was an NHS bed available locally, it could not be used due to staff leaving and not being allowed to be replaced.

We have worked hard to try to develop a true partnership with the provider arm of our local primary care trust, and although relationships are generally very positive, it has been impossible to translate words into action. We have spent a great deal of time in meetings with senior managers and clinicians, talking about developing joint services, removing duplication, making joint appointments, merging consultant on-call rotas and sharing Mental Health Act support. Unfortunately, this had led to nothing other than frustration on our part, and we are left with the impression that we, and the whole of the independent sector, are viewed as a necessary evil only to be used as a very last resort. All of the above ideas would have offered opportunities to improve quality and to save costs, and it is hard to see why a financially challenged PCT should wish to reject them so quickly.

Our progress with the commissioning arm of the PCT has been similarly frustrating. Whilst they report very positively on our service, a commissioning document that we have seen states quite clearly that the independent sector should only be used when no NHS bed is available, regardless of the type of referral. This is disheartening and seems somewhat at odds with the plurality and patient-choice agendas.

THE INDEPENDENT SECTOR IN GENERAL

Typically, other independent providers have also gone down the route of developing specialist services, many of them having chosen psychiatric intensive care units or some other type of low- or medium-security provision. Many feel that they are seen as providers of last resort and that commissioning of their services is often a stopgap measure rather than being part of a longer-term contract. This is a missed opportunity for all parties, as it prevents the independent-sector providers from being able to plan on any long-term basis and also means that the NHS is unable to benefit fully from the negotiation of discounts for bulk contracting.

The independent sector is generally experiencing a downturn in referrals for all types of services because of the financial position across the NHS. While there are indications of some creative approaches towards commissioning – where groups of commissioners together form consortia in order to negotiate better prices – there are worrying indications elsewhere. For example, the reduction in referrals of patients with brain injury means that some such patients are not getting the help they require; we are aware that some are even being discharged home without rehabilitation care.

Many independent providers, including The Retreat, suffered as a result of the Care Standards Act 2000, when they were obliged to change their registration status from that of a mental nursing home to an independent hospital, in order to continue to admit individuals detained under the Mental Health Act. This led to an increased exposure to value-added tax on capital upgrades and developments, to the removal of free access to general medical services and NHS prescriptions and to problems with local-authority funding. Such difficulties seem not to have been an intended outcome of the new legislation but rather are an unfortunate consequence of something that had not been properly thought through. Among other negative impacts of the legislation upon the sector are an increase in the cost base and a great deal of additional work with no tangible benefits to service users – and that is without mentioning the whole gamut of new costs following the inception of the Healthcare Commission and the Criminal Records Bureau.

Another major cost pressure for the independent sector is that of employment costs, which have risen inexorably over the past few years. Although many in the sector steer away from direct links with NHS pay rates, particularly Agenda for Change, we all recognise that we are competing for the same pool of staff and that our rates need to be comparable with those offered by the NHS. However, pay itself is not really the issue: the independent sector recognises the need to offer an attractive salary in order to attract and retain the highest calibre of staff and is often able to pay higher rates than those on offer in the NHS. The problems come, rather, with the other conditions of service, namely pension, sick pay and holidays and access to training.

Many independent-sector organisations have never had any sort of final salary pension scheme, offering only a defined contribution scheme. A good number of those who have offered a final salary scheme have needed to review and amend it, often significantly, because they have recognised that it is simply not affordable. In our sector we all know that a pension scheme can

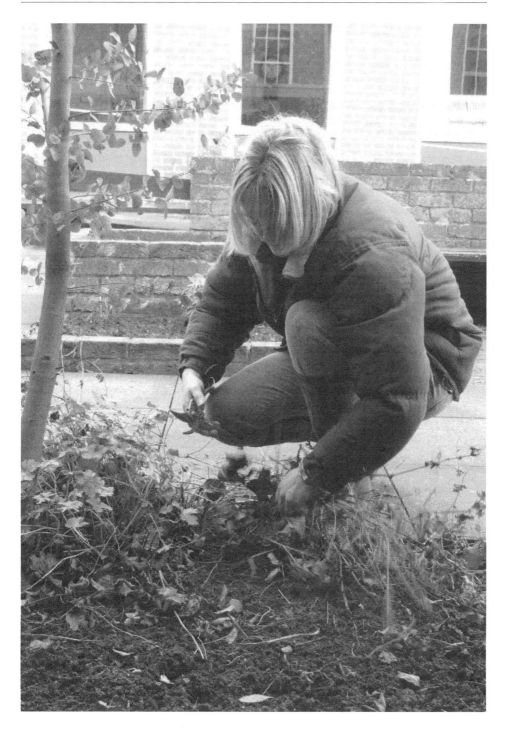

FIGURE 15.2 Horticulture therapy at The Retreat, York. Reproduced with kind permission.

bring about the demise of an organisation and we are unwilling to take that risk. We continue to look disbelievingly across at the final salary, index-linked NHS pension scheme which, looking to the future, is unaffordable and yet is still retained.

The story with sick-pay entitlements is similar, and much benefit could surely be gained by rewarding more handsomely those who come to work rather than those who don't. I know some independent-sector organisations which have implemented a discretionary sick-pay scheme, although we have not yet done that at The Retreat.

With regard to training and development, it has been our experience that some staff are turning down positions with us because the NHS has offered them a post which includes one day off a week to pursue a course, sometimes apparently unconnected with their role. We, like other independent-sector organisations, have a good track record in supporting training and development but it has to be linked to the needs of the service as well as to those of the individual, so funding and time off are carefully negotiated. If everyone spent 20% of their time on training, we would simply be unable to survive.

THE FUTURE

Looking ahead, the rhetoric would indicate that there are many opportunities for the independent sector, primarily as a result of the increased emphasis on the split between commissioning and providing, and the recognition of the complementary roles of different providers ('pluralities'). Indeed, we are starting to see references to the independent sector and its important role in the market-place, and some small examples are coming to light of PCTs stipulating a minimum non-NHS component to certain elements of their commissioning. Patient choice adds to this, as service users generally speak very highly of the independent sector, partly as a result of our strong focus on customer care which not all NHS services seem able to match.

The advent of Foundation Trusts and their description as independent providers, rather than part of the NHS, should lead to an opening up of the market and a greater acceptance of the role of independent providers in their broadest sense. In many ways the independent sector ought to be ahead of the game in this type of market, as we are already experienced in the need to sell our services. As commissioners grow into their role, there should be the chance for independent providers to bid for whole service systems and to emphasise the value for money we have to offer. Such bids may be made individually or in partnership with other NHS or non-NHS organisations. If independent providers are successful, this could lead to our providing not just specialist mental health services but also more routine services. The introduction of Payment by Results offers the independent sector the opportunity to debunk the myth that it is expensive and to show that we can offer a high-quality service that meets the needs of service users and represents clear value for money.

On the other hand, there is still strong evidence that the importance of plurality has not yet been fully embraced by those making decisions at local level, as evidenced by using the independent sector as a provider of last resort. There is therefore a risk that the opportunities will not come soon enough and that some organisations will not survive. There is much talk of our 'battening down the hatches' and 'riding out the storm' for the next twelve to eighteen months, but that requires healthy reserves if you are a charity or patient investors if you are a commercial company. Not all organisations find themselves in such a position.

Even if the opportunities do materialise, the NHS will, undoubtedly, become more business-like in its commissioning and there will be greater competition for those high-cost, low-volume specialist services that have traditionally been provided by the independent sector. This increased competition and more openness about costings will mean an end to the super profits that some independents have been able to access by providing some of these specialist services.

The NHS will become better equipped to market its services using quality and outcome measures and will also be more active in recruitment and retention incentives, all of which will put further pressures on the independent sector. One need only look at the boards of Foundation Trusts to see that changes are afoot; board members increasingly possess strong commercial backgrounds and are collectively likely to take a more aggressive, business-like approach to managing costs than has existed in the past.

Will the opportunities outweigh the threats? I have always believed that the NHS could solve its financial difficulties if it mirrored a public limited company (plc) and started to function as one head office with a number of subsidiary companies. This would result in handsome economies of scale and in the various components working with rather than against one another. Even if that were not possible on a national level, it should be so at strategic health authority level, with all players focusing on a single health community, rationalising services, releasing estate to develop new services in-house and sharing support services. However, I believe that such an outcome is unlikely in the short term, as the concept of NHS plc as yet finds no resonance and cross-boundary thinking remains comparatively underdeveloped.

Indeed, government policy is leading the NHS in the opposite direction, towards an open and competitive market where Foundation Trusts are being set apart from other sections of the NHS. I believe that this will increase the tendency to think in silos and leave the independent sector with new opportunities for expansion, particularly once more effective commissioning gets off the ground and existing providers remain preoccupied with mergers and re-structuring.

REFERENCES

1 Porter R. *Mind-Forg'd Manacles*. 2nd ed. London: Penguin; 1990.
2 Tuke S. *Description of The Retreat*. 2nd ed. London: Process Press; 1996.

Index